Keto Diet Cookbook for Beginners

Easy, Quick and Delicious Ketogenic Diet Recipes For Busy People | Eat Healthy and Lose Weight Fast!

Table of Contents

INTRODUCTION 6
WHAT IS KETOGENIC DIET? 7
What can I eat on keto? 8
What can't I eat on keto? 11
KETOGENIC RECIPES 13
About these recipes 13
Breakfast 15
    Eggs, Bacon, Spinach and Mushroom Bowls 16
    Avocado, Coconut Oil and Chia Seed Smoothie 17
    Keto Protein Pancakes 18
    Salmon and Avocado Stack with Garlic Spinach 19
    Raspberry Almond Overnight "Oats" 20
    Chocolate Strawberry Pancakes 21
    Egg, Turkey and Chive Muffins 22
    Keto Cinnamon Roll Granola 23
    Blueberry and almond fat-bomb smoothie 24
    Fat-Dense Iced Coffee Shake 25
    Scrambled Eggs with "Green Sauce" 26
Meat mains 28
    Pan-Fried Steaks with Sour Cream Mushroom Sauce 29
    Spiced Lamb and Pepper Skewers 30
    Beef Stroganoff with Buttered Zoodles 31
    Venison Winter Pie 32
    Beef and Bacon Meatballs 34
    Parmesan and Sunflower Seed Beef Patties 35
    Eggplant, Beef and Mozzarella Bake 36
    Ginger and Garlic Pork Stir Fry 37
    Beef Taco Cowls 38
    Rich Lamb Bolognese 39
    Beef and Peanut Curry 40
    Slow-Cooked Pulled Pork with Spices 42
    Fresh Beef Salad 43
Fish mains 44
    Pan-Seared Fresh White Fish with Butter, Lemon and Parsley ... 45
    Smoked Salmon and Cream Cheese Dip with Lemon Zest 46
    Oven-Baked Fish with Tomatoes and Herbs 47

Simple Fish Stir Fry with Sesame Seeds and Scallions 48
Fish Taco Bowls 49
Parmesan Crusted Fish 50
Tuna Cakes 51
Fish with Capers, Cream, Lemon and Wine 52
Fish and Eggplant Curry (Mild and Creamy) 53
Fish Skewers with Lemon Mayo 54
Raw Fish Platter with Wasabi Cream 55
Chili Prawn Salad 56
Seared Scallops with Wine and Cream Sauce (Special Occasion Recipe for Guests) 57
Prawn and Chorizo Stir Fry with Fresh Herbs and Parmesan 58

Chicken Dishes 59

Oven-Baked Drumsticks with Sesame Seeds 60
Chicken Thighs with Sun Dried Tomato Cream Sauce 61
Chicken Stir Fry with Orange and Scallions 62
Chicken and Mozzarella Patties 63
Chicken, Broccoli and Cashew Stir Fry 64
Whole Roasted Chicken with Roasted Cauliflower 65
Chicken Wings with Chili-Lime Aioli 66
Chicken, Mushroom and Leek Stew 67
Chicken, Feta and Olive Salad 68
Slow-Cooked Chicken Chili 69
Chicken and Tomato Tray Bake 70
Chicken and Bell Pepper Fajitas 71
Chicken and Avocado Sushi 72

Loaded Keto Smoothies 73

Avocado and Strawberry Smoothie 74
Cinnamon Bun Smoothie 75
Super Green Smoothie 76
Chocolate Raspberry Smoothie 77
Peanut Butter and Jam Smoothie 78
Wake-Me-Up Coffee Smoothie 79
Berries and Cream Smoothie 80
Mint Choc Chip Smoothie 81
Mango, Spinach and Strawberry Smoothie 82
Creamy Chia and Vanilla Smoothie 83
Coconut and Lime Smoothie 84
Blueberry and Almond Butter Smoothie 85
Halloween Pumpkin Spice Smoothie 86

Sweet Treats, Desserts and Sweet Drinks **87**
    Chocolate Truffles 88
    Peanut Butter Fat Bombs 89
    Berries and Cream Pots 90
    Coconut Berry Ice Cream 91
    Vanilla Choc Chip Ice Cream..92
    Almond and Peanut Butter Chocolate Cookie Bites 93
    Chocolate Avocado Mousse 94
    Coconut Vanilla Latte..95
    Peppermint Hot Chocolate...96
    Lemon Cream 97
    Sweet and Creamy Chai Latte 98
    Chili Spice Hot Chocolate...99
CONCLUSION **100**

Introduction

Hey there! Welcome and come on in! You've arrived at the best place to be if you're just starting out on the ketogenic diet. Here we will talk about the benefits of the ketogenic diet, what you can and can't eat, and of course...we've got a whole set of delicious recipes! These recipes are really easy to make and involve ingredients which are easy to source and won't cost you an arm and a leg. Each recipe has been designed with time-consciousness in mind, because I know that you're a busy guy or gal who doesn't have time for dilly dallying for hours in the kitchen. You can fit these recipes into your busy week filled with family, work and friends. And most importantly, each recipe has been calculated according to the macronutrient-based rules of the ketogenic diet so you can be confident as you nibble away!

I am sure you are already clued-up about the ketogenic diet, but I'm here to give you a refresher! Whether you're doing the ketogenic diet for weight loss, extra energy, mental clarity or to reduce your risk of disease, your body will certainly thank you...and so will your tastebuds.

But enough of this chit chat! Let's get into the nitty gritty of the ketogenic diet...

What Is Ketogenic Diet?

The ketogenic diet is a strict eating plan which is entirely based on macronutrients: fat, protein and carbohydrates. The idea is to heavily reduce your carbohydrate intake, increase your fat intake and keep your protein intake moderate. When you cut out most carbohydrates and sugars, your body responds by tapping into your fat stores for energy, as well as releasing ketone bodies for energy, aka "ketosis". This leads to fat loss, stabilized blood sugar levels, more energy and a clearer head!

Historically, the ketogenic diet was first prescribed by doctors for patients who were suffering from epilepsy. In fact, the ketogenic diet is a type of fasting, which has been practised for millenia!

Many people find that by cutting out carbohydrates and sugars, they are cutting out foods which make them sick, sluggish and tired. Foods such as processed bread, baked goods, candy, sugary drinks and fried fast foods are all banned on keto, and should be replaced with fresh veggies, meats, full-fat dairy, seeds and nuts. This change naturally leads to more energy because there are simply more nutrients in these keto-approved foods. You'll also find that your calorie intake naturally reduces too, resulting in weight loss and healthier measurements (woohoo! New clothes!).

The bottom line? The ketogenic diet is a very low carb and high fat diet which is popular for weight loss, energy levels, blood sugar issues and overall good health.

I must be a bit of a worry-wart for a moment and just make sure that you are taking care of your health safely. For that reason, I'll just mention here that it's always very important to see your doctor before drastically changing your diet, especially if you are pregnant, breastfeeding, trying to conceive, or have pre-existing health issues. But that's all I'll say on the matter!

Let's talk about food...

What can I eat on keto?

On the ketogenic diet you can expect to eat a diet full of: fresh, non-starchy veggies, a few berries (in moderation), nuts, seeds, oils, butter, cream, full-fat dairy, coconut cream, grass-fed beef, free range chicken, wild-caught fish, nut butters, and natural sweeteners such as stevia. And of course, you can use little amounts of spices and lots of fresh herbs too.

THE YES LIST:

Green, non-starchy veggies such as:
- Broccoli
- Lettuces
- Spinach
- Kale
- Celery
- Cucumber

Other veggies such as:
- Eggplant
- Bell peppers
- Tomatoes
- Garlic (small amounts)
- Onion (tiny amounts)

Berries in small amounts
- Blueberries
- Strawberries
- Raspberries
- Boysenberries
- *Citrus in small amounts*
- Juice and zest of lemon, lime and orange (small amounts!)

Full-fat dairy
- Butter
- Cream
- Full-fat Greek yogurt

Grass-fed meats
- Beef
- Lamb

- Venison
- Ground red meats

Free-range chicken
- Whole chicken
- Breast
- Thigh
- Wings
- Drumsticks
- Ground chicken

Wild-caught fish
- Salmon
- Tuna
- White fish (i.e. snapper)

Free-range eggs

Nuts
- Almonds
- Walnuts
- Pecans
- Brazil nuts
- Peanuts (small amounts)

Seeds
- Sesame seeds
- Chia seeds
- Pumpkin seeds
- Sunflower seeds

Oils
- Olive
- Avocado
- Coconut
- Flaxseed
- Peanut
- Sesame

Extras
- Coconut cream

- Almond milk
- Nut butters
- Tamari soy sauce
- Mayonnaise
- Aioli
- Fish sauce
- 72% cocoa dark chocolate

Alcohol
- Small amounts of wine and spirits with zero-carb, zero-sugar mixers such as plain sparkling water

What can't I eat on keto?

On the ketogenic diet it's crucial that you stay away from high-carb, high-sugar foods such as: breads, pasta, rice, potatoes, sweet potatoes, sugar, honey, lentils, beans, chickpeas, candy, sugary drinks...you'll get the hang of it! It actually starts to become very intuitive after a while. However, it's important to use your macro counter (i.e. MyFitnessPal) religiously at the start because there are many products which have unexpected hidden carbs and sugars. For that reason, it's best to stick with whole foods, straight from the source because that way, you know exactly what you are eating.

THE NO LIST

Baked goods (unless they're certified keto-friendly!)
- Breads
- Cakes
- Pastries
- Cookies
- Bars
- Sugary desserts

Candy
- All candy unless it specifically states that it is "keto approved"

Starchy veggies
- Peas
- Potatoes
- Sweet potato
- Parsnip
- Corn
- Squash

Grains and starches
- Pasta
- All rice
- Polenta
- Couscous
- Oats
- Barley
- Quinoa

Legumes and pulses
- All bens (i.e. kidney beans, black beans, cannellini beans)
- All lentils
- Chickpeas

Sugary drinks
- Sodas
- Fruit juices
- Sugary pre-mixed alcoholic drinks

Milk (stick to cream)

Ketogenic recipes

About these recipes

Serves

Each recipe has a "serves" at the start, followed by a number. This tells you how many servings the recipe yields. The nutritional information has been calculated per single serving. You might find that you would like a larger or smaller serving size than what the recipe states, but you can simply use the nutritional information as a guide and shuffle it around according to how many servings you get out of the recipe.

Time

The "time" section of each recipe is an approximate time which lets you know how long to allow yourself to create the recipe. Everyone's cooking style and pace is different, so take this as a guess!

Ingredients

The ingredients lists are set out with US measurements to let you know exactly how much of everything you need. Certain ingredients such as salt, pepper and oil may not have a measurement before them. In the case of salt and pepper, it simply means to use a sprinkle to taste. Taste your dish then add more salt and pepper accordingly. It's amazing how different people's taste buds are when it comes to salt! Where it says "a drizzle" of olive oil, it simply means a quick slosh in a pan...about a tablespoon if you must measure.

Just a note on garlic: many of the savory recipes in this book feature garlic powder. This is because it's so much easier to sprinkle garlic powder over your dish than it is to peel and chopped garlic cloves! Some recipes do use fresh garlic cloves, but otherwise we just stick to the handy old powder!

Method

The method is set out in numbered form, with each step clearly and easily explained so you can cook with ease!

Nutritional information

At the end of each recipe, you'll find the nutritional information in this format:
Calories:
Fat:
Protein:
Total carbs:
Net carbs:

This information refers to *each serving*. This way, you know *exactly* how many calories you are eating, but more importantly, how many carbs, fats and proteins. The "total carbs" refers to the carbs including the fiber. The "net carbs" refers to the carbs *minus* the fiber, and it's the most important number to be aware of. Most people aim for a net carb intake of around 20 grams per day.

Breakfast

I know what you might be thinking, "I'm not a big breakfast eater"...but don't skip this section! Even if eating in the morning is a chore for you, give it a try, even if it's just a fat-filled smoothie or a little nibble of keto granola or a light egg muffin. In this section, you will find breakfast recipes for rushed early mornings, leisurely weekend mid-mornings and everything in between. Lots of eggs, oils, bacon, cheese, seeds, avocado, berries and fresh veggies await.

Eggs, Bacon, Spinach and Mushroom Bowls

The reason I call these "bowls" is because you fry everything together and (lovingly) toss it all into a bowl to eat easily with nothing but a fork, as opposed to laying it on a plate to eat with a set of cutlery. You've got protein, lots of fats, fiber and green veggie goodness all in one bowl.

Serves: 2
Time: approximately 20 minutes
Ingredients:
- 2 Tbsp olive oil
- 6 bacon rashers, roughly chopped
- 1 ½ cups sliced mushrooms
- 2 cups chopped fresh spinach
- 4 eggs, lightly beaten
- Salt and pepper
- 1 tsp garlic powder

Method:
1. Drizzle the olive oil into a non-stick frying pan and place it over a medium heat
2. Add the bacon and sizzle until the pieces release their fat and become crispy
3. Add the mushrooms and stir to coat in the bacon fat, allow them to soften and become slightly brown
4. Add the spinach and stir to coat in the fats and oils, heat until the spinach wilts
5. Move the bacon and veggies to the side of the frying pan to make room for the eggs
6. Add the eggs to the pan and sprinkle with salt, pepper and garlic salt before moving them around with a wooden spoon as they lightly scramble. As long as they're cooked there's no rules, they don't need to be perfect!
7. Divide everything evenly between two bowls and serve right away!

Nutritional information:
- **Calories:** 480
- **Fat:** 38 grams
- **Protein:** 26.1 grams
- **Total carbs:** 4.4 grams
- **Net carbs:** 2.3 grams

Avocado, Coconut Oil and Chia Seed Smoothie

This smoothie is very rich in fat and fiber, meaning it will keep you fueled and full until lunchtime or even later. The healthy fats in the avocado, chia seeds and coconut oil are great for fat burning but they're also wonderful for soft, soothed and young-looking skin (yay! Bonus!).

Serves: 2
Time: 10 minutes
Ingredients:
- 2 avocados
- 3 Tbsp coconut oil (melted if your oil has solidified)
- 3 Tbsp chia seeds, hydrated in 6 Tbsp of water for 5 minutes
- 2 cups unsweetened almond milk
- Few drops of stevia to taste
- 2 handfuls of ice

Method:
1. Place all ingredients into a blender and blitz until extra smooth
2. Serve right away to make sure the smoothie stays cool and creamy

Nutritional information:
Calories: 534
Fat: 49 grams
Protein: 8.4 grams
Total carbs: 20.5
Net carbs: 2 grams (yup, lots of fiber in this smoothie!)

Keto Protein Pancakes

These pancakes are fluffy, soft and filling. They're made mainly from eggs, protein powder and almond flour. Use a natural, unsweetened whey protein powder. Top them with a little squeeze of lemon juice.

Serves: 2
Time: approximately 25 minutes
Ingredients:

- 4 eggs
- 2 scoops plain whey protein (or pea protein for vegans)
- 4 Tbsp almond flour
- 1 tsp baking powder
- 1 tsp vanilla extract
- Coconut oil for frying
- Juice of 1 lemon

Method:

1. Whisk together the eggs, protein powder, almond flour, baking powder and vanilla extract until combined and smooth
2. Place a non-stick frying pan over a medium-high heat
3. Add a little drizzle of oil to the pan
4. When the pan is nice and hot, add a spoonful of pancake mixture
5. Once you see bubbles appearing on the pancake, flip it over to cook the other side
6. Repeat until you've cooked all of the mixture and you have a pile of hot, fluffy pancakes
7. Divide the pancakes between two plates and drizzle with lemon juice
8. Serve!

Nutritional information:

- **Calories:** 351
- **Fat:** 23.2 grams
- **Protein:** 25.2 grams
- **Total carbs:** 12.9 grams
- **Net carbs:** 6.9 grams

Salmon and Avocado Stack with Garlic Spinach

Salmon and avocado provide excellent fats to keep you full and help that keto process run smoothly, they're also wonderful for soothing inflamed skin and helping to prevent signs of aging. Garlic spinach adds those crucial leafy greens to our morning.

Serves: 2
Time: 10 minutes
Ingredients:

- 4 oz hot smoked salmon, flaked into chunks
- 2 avocados, sliced
- 2 Tbsp olive oil
- 1 Tbsp butter
- 2 garlic cloves, finely chopped
- 4 cups spinach (it wilts down!)
- Salt and pepper

Method:

1. Lay a few avocado slices down onto each serving plate (2 plates), then add a few salmon chunks, lay over another avocado slice, then repeat the process so you have two even stacks, set aside
2. Add the oil and butter to a frying pan and place over a medium heat
3. When the butter has melted, add the garlic to the pan and allow to soften but not brown
4. Add the spinach and stir to coat in oil and butter, stir as it completely wilts
5. Divide the spinach between the two plates, next to the avocado salmon stacks
6. Serve immediately!

Nutritional information:

- **Calories:** 590
- **Fat:** 53.8 grams
- **Protein:** 15.8 grams
- **Total carbs:** 15.1 grams
- **Net carbs:** 3.6 grams

Raspberry Almond Overnight "Oats"

This is not really an oat dish...but it's a keto take on the popular overnight oat breakfast dish. We use chia seeds, LSA meal (linseed, sunflower seed and almond mix), pumpkin seeds and almonds. Lots of fiber, lots of fat! For the raspberries, we use freeze dried raspberry powder because it brings the tasty flavor without the added carbs.

Serves: 2
Time: overnight
Ingredients:
- 3 Tbsp chia seeds
- 3 Tbsp LSA meal
- 2 Tbsp pumpkin seeds
- 4 Tbsp ground almonds
- 3 Tbsp coconut thread (unsweetened)
- 2 Tbsp freeze dried raspberry powder
- 1 tsp vanilla extract
- 1 ½ cups unsweetened almond milk

Method:
1. Mix together all of the ingredients in a bowl then divide between two serving bowls
2. Cover and store in the fridge overnight
3. In the morning, give it a good stir. If it's a little too thick you can add a dash of water or more almond milk
4. Enjoy!

Nutritional information:
- **Calories:** 380
- **Fat:** 27.7 grams
- **Protein:** 14.4 grams
- **Total carbs:** 20.7 grams
- **Net carbs:** 4.5 grams

Chocolate Strawberry Pancakes

Sweet, chocolatey, strawberry pancakes! These are super easy and can be whipped up in your blender. Serve with a few slices of fresh strawberry and some whipped cream for a decadent treat.

Serves: 2
Time: approximately 25 minutes
Ingredients:
- 4 eggs
- 2 Tbsp unsweetened cocoa powder
- 3 Tbsp ground almonds
- 4 large strawberries
- 1 tsp baking powder
- Pinch of salt

To cook:
- Coconut oil

To serve:
- 2 strawberries, sliced (1 strawberry per serving)
- ½ cup heavy whipping cream, whipped
- Drop of stevia to sweeten the cream

Method:
1. Place the eggs, cocoa, ground almonds, strawberries, baking powder and salt into your blender and blitz until totally smooth
2. Place a non-stick frying pan over a medium heat and add a drizzle of coconut oil
3. Pour dollops of batter onto the hot frying pan and cook on both sides (you'll know when it's time to flip the pancakes when bubbles appear on the top)
4. Serve each stack of pancakes with a sliced strawberry and a dollop of whipped cream

Nutritional information:
- **Calories:** 219
- **Fat:** 15.1 grams
- **Protein:** 15.7 grams
- **Total carbs:** 7.7 grams
- **Net carbs:** 4.2 grams

Egg, Turkey and Chive Muffins

These muffins are like a muffin and a quiche had a baby! No flour in sight, just fats and proteins and veggies. You can substitute turkey for chicken, but I love turkey for a change. Lots of cheese, chives and eggy goodness awaits for a quick, on-the-run breakfast.

Serves: makes 12 muffins (1 muffin per serving)
Time: approximately 25 minutes
Ingredients:

- 8 eggs, lightly beaten
- ½ cup heavy cream
- 10 oz shredded cooked turkey meat
- ½ cup finely chopped fresh chives
- 1 cup grated cheddar cheese
- 1 cup shredded spinach
- 6 oz cream cheese, cut into small pieces
- Salt and pepper

Method:

1. Preheat the oven to 350 degrees Fahrenheit and grease a 12-hole muffin pan with butter or oil
2. Whisk together the eggs and cream in a large bowl, preferably one with a pouring spout
3. Add the rest of the ingredients and stir to combine
4. Divide the mixture between your greased muffin holes
5. Place into the oven and bake for about 15 minutes or until just set but still very slightly wobbly in the middle
6. Leave to cool before turning out and placing in an airtight container
7. Store in the fridge!

Nutritional information:

- **Calories:** 157
- **Fat:** 10.6 grams
- **Protein:** 9.5 grams
- **Total carbs:** 1.1 grams
- **Net carbs:** 1.1 grams

Keto Cinnamon Roll Granola

This granola is really a delicious combination of seeds, nuts, nut flours, spices and keto-friendly natural sweeteners. It's amazing sprinkled over full-fat yogurt in the morning, with a drizzle of flaxseed oil for extra fats.

Serves: makes 5 servings
Time: approximately 20 minutes
Ingredients:
- 4 Tbsp coconut oil
- 1 cup almond flour
- ⅓ cup slivered almonds
- ⅓ cup chopped walnuts
- ⅓ cup desiccated coconut
- 3 Tbsp chia seeds
- 2 Tbsp flaxseed
- 4 Tbsp pumpkin seeds
- 2 tsp ground cinnamon mixed with powdered stevia to taste
- Pinch of salt

Method:
1. Place a very large sauté pan over a medium heat and add the coconut oil to the pan
2. Add all of the remaining ingredients to the hot pan (yup, just toss them all in!) and stir to combine
3. Keep stirring as the granola gently toasts
4. Give it a taste and test the sweetness, if it's not sweet enough, add more stevia
5. Leave to cool completely before transferring into an airtight container and storing in a cool place

Nutritional information:
- **Calories:** 443
- **Fat:** 41.2 grams
- **Protein:** 12.2 grams
- **Total carbs:** 12.5 grams
- **Net carbs:** 3.7 grams

Blueberry and almond fat-bomb smoothie

Sometimes you just want a delicious, cold smoothie to sip on in the morning, and this one here is a real winner. Blueberries are a tasty source of antioxidants, with almond milk providing low-carb creaminess, and flaxseed oil adding healthy, skin-nourishing fats.

Serves: 2
Time: 5 minutes
Ingredients:

- ½ cup blueberries
- 1 ½ cups unsweetened almond milk
- 2 Tbsp flaxseed oil
- 1 avocado (we use this as a banana replacement for creaminess and thickness)
- Handful of ice
- Few drops of stevia to taste

Method:

1. Place all ingredients into a blender and blitz until velvety smooth
2. Give the smoothie a taste and add more stevia if it's not sweet enough for your liking
3. Pour and sip immediately

Nutritional information:

- **Calories:** 281
- **Fat:** 26.5 grams
- **Protein:** 2.5 grams
- **Total carbs:** 12 grams
- **Net carbs:** 5 grams

Fat-Dense Iced Coffee Shake

Another smoothie! This time it's spiked with coffee...you're welcome. Double your breakfast with your morning caffeine hit...time-saving and delicious.

Serves: 2
Time: 5 minutes
Ingredients:
- 2 tsp espresso powder, dissolved in 2 Tbsp hot water
- ¾ cup heavy cream
- 1 ½ cups unsweetened almond milk
- 2 Tbsp MCT oil or coconut oil
- 2 large handfuls of ice
- Liquid stevia to taste

Method:
1. Place all ingredients into a blender and blitz until slushy and thick
2. Taste for sweetness and add more stevia if need be
3. Enjoy right away, before the ice melts

Nutritional information:
- **Calories:** 456
- **Fat:** 49 grams
- **Protein:** 2.5 grams
- **Total carbs:** 3.7 grams
- **Net carbs:** 2.9 grams

Scrambled Eggs with "Green Sauce"

Scrambled eggs are a breakfast classic, and they're completely keto-approved. But to increase the nutritional profile of this breakfast, we add a "green sauce", made from herbs, olive oil, garlic, parmesan and spinach.

Serves: 2
Time: approximately 20 minutes
Ingredients:
- 1 tsp butter
- 4 eggs
- 4 Tbsp heavy cream
- ⅓ cup grated cheese (I use colby but you can use your favorite)
- Salt and pepper

Sauce:
- Handful of fresh parsley
- Handful of fresh basil
- Few fresh mint leaves
- 1 cup fresh spinach
- 3 Tbsp pine nuts
- ½ fresh garlic clove
- ⅓ cup grated parmesan cheese
- Juice of ½ lemon
- Salt and pepper

Method:
1. Place all of the sauce ingredients into a small blender or food processor and pulse until combined and smooth. It's okay for there to be a few smaller chunks, but mostly smooth, set aside
2. Place a non-stick frying pan over a medium heat and add the butter to the pan, allow it to melt while you prepare the eggs
3. Whisk together the eggs, cream, cheese, salt and pepper
4. Pour the egg/cheese mixture into the hot frying pan and use a wooden spatula to "nudge" the eggs around the pan. A good method is to drag the spatula through the eggs from the sides to the center to allow the eggs to scramble and cook evenly without turning into an omelet
5. Divide the eggs between two plates and drizzle a spoonful of green sauce over the top
6. Store leftover green sauce in an airtight container in the fridge

Nutritional information:

- **Calories:** 486
- **Fat:** 36.8 grams
- **Protein:** 23.3 grams
- **Total carbs:** 5.6 grams
- **Net carbs:** 4.8 grams

Meat mains

Now we come to the meatiest section in the book! This section is dedicated to meat-based dishes to serve at dinner time or for a very special lunch. We've got beef steaks, lamb, venison, pork and ground meats to make your mouth water. Remember to buy grass-fed meats from ethical sources.

Pan-Fried Steaks with Sour Cream Mushroom Sauce

Beef steaks cooked on a hot skillet and doused in creamy mushroom sauce...impressive, right? But it's also super easy to prepare and is doable for even the most nervous of cooks.

Serves: 4
Time: approximately 30 minutes
Ingredients:
- 4 (4 oz) beef steaks
- 2 Tbsp olive oil
- 2 Tbsp butter
- 2 garlic cloves, finely chopped
- 2 ½ cups sliced mushrooms (I like to use a mixture of portobello and button mushrooms)
- ½ cup dry white wine
- ½ cup sour cream
- ½ cup heavy cream
- Salt and pepper

Method:
1. Make sure the beef steaks are at room temperature so take them out of the fridge an hour before you start cooking
2. Drizzle the olive oil into a sauté pan and add the butter, place the pan over a medium-high heat and allow the butter and oil to melt together and become hot
3. Add the garlic and soften for a minute or two
4. Add the mushrooms and stir as they soften and brown
5. Add the wine and allow it to simmer so the alcohol "burns off", about 5 minutes
6. Add the cream, sour cream, salt and pepper, turn the heat down to low and allow the sauce to simmer and thicken as you cook the steaks
7. Rub the steaks with olive oil and sprinkle each side with salt and pepper
8. Place a skillet over a high heat and wait for it to become nice and hot
9. Add the steaks to the hot skillet and cook on both sides until you reach your desired doneness (medium rare is my preference)
10. Serve the steaks with a generous spoon of mushroom sauce over top

Nutritional information:
- **Calories:** 519
- **Fat:** 37.5 grams
- **Protein:** 35.6 grams
- **Total carbs:** 4.4 grams
- **Net carbs:** 3.7 grams

Spiced Lamb and Pepper Skewers

A super easy supper with lamb and bell peppers threaded onto skewers and grilled to perfection! Serve with a salad or simply nibble on a couple for a light lunch or barbeque starter.

Serves: 6 (makes 12 skewers, 2 skewers per serving)
Time: approximately 30 minutes
Ingredients:
- 2 lb lamb, cubed
- 4 large bell peppers (variety of colors), seeds and core removed, flesh cut into chunks to match the size of the lamb
- 4 Tbsp olive oil
- Salt and pepper

Method:
1. Thread the lamb and bell pepper chunks onto your skewers, but make sure to leave room on either side so you can pick the skewers up easily
2. Rub the lamb and peppers with olive oil, salt and pepper
3. Place a skillet over a high heat
4. Place the filled skewers onto the hot skillet and turn to allow each side to become charred
5. The lamb should be cooked but still "blushing" inside
6. Pile onto a platter and serve!

Serving suggestions: make a homemade pesto to drizzle over each skewer. Serve over a bed of cauliflower rice.

Nutritional information:
- **Calories:** 474
- **Fat:** 36.6 grams
- **Protein:** 32.4 grams
- **Total carbs:** 4 grams
- **Net carbs:** 2.7 grams

Beef Stroganoff with Buttered Zoodles

This is a simplified version of beef stroganoff anyone can make! We serve it with zucchini noodles which have been tossed in melted butter. A comforting dish any keto newbie will love.

Serves: 4
Time: approximately 40 minutes
Ingredients:
- 4 Tbsp olive oil
- 1 ½ lbs beef strips
- 2 garlic cloves, finely chopped
- 2 cups button mushrooms, sliced
- 1 Tbsp tomato paste
- 1 cup beef stock
- 1 cup sour cream
- Salt and pepper
- 2 large zucchinis, cut into noodles using a spiralizer, food processor or knife
- 3 Tbsp butter, melted
- Salt and pepper

Method:
1. Drizzle the olive oil into a large sauté pan and place over a medium-high heat
2. Add the beef strips and garlic to the pan and stir for a few minutes to allow the beef to brown
3. Add the mushrooms and stir for a couple of minutes to allow them to soften
4. Add the tomato paste and stir into the beef and mushrooms
5. Add the beef stock, sour cream, salt and pepper and reduce the heat to allow the stroganoff to simmer and thicken as you prep the zucchini noodles
6. Place the zucchini noodles into a microwave-safe bowl and blast in the microwave on high for 2 minutes before pouring the melted butter over top and tossing to coat
7. Serve the stroganoff hot, over a pile of hot buttered zoodles!

Nutritional information:
- **Calories:** 676
- **Fat:** 46 grams
- **Protein:** 53.4 grams
- **Total carbs:** 8.5 grams
- **Net carbs:** 6.8 grams

Venison Winter Pie

Have you ever cooked with venison? It's a rich meat which does really well when slow cooked to tender perfection. We combine venison meat with bacon, stock and herbs, pour it into a pie dish and top it with mashed cauliflower. Something a little different to experiment with!

Serves: 6
Time: approximately 4 hours
Ingredients:
- 4 Tbsp olive oil
- ½ onion, finely chopped
- 4 garlic cloves, finely chopped
- 6 bacon rashers, chopped into little pieces (no need to be exact, just chop them roughly!)
- 2 lb venison meat cubes
- 1 tsp dried rosemary
- 1 tsp dried thyme
- 2 cups beef stock
- ½ cup red wine
- Salt and pepper
- 1 cauliflower head, cut into florets
- ½ cup cream
- 3 Tbsp butter
- Salt and pepper

Method:
1. Drizzle the olive oil into your slow cooker or Dutch oven and set to a medium-high heat
2. Add the onion, garlic and bacon and sizzle until the bacon is cooked and the onions are soft
3. Add the venison meat and toss as it browns
4. Add the herbs, stock, wine, salt and pepper, stir to combine before placing the lid onto the pot
5. If you're using a slow cooker, set to *high* temperature for four hours. If using the oven, cook for four hours at 380 degrees Fahrenheit
6. Check the venison every once in a while and if it's starting to become dry, add a little more stock (unlikely, but good to know!)
7. Place the cauliflower florets into a steamer over a pot of boiling water and cover, steam until the florets are soft

8. Add the cooked cauliflower into a blender and add the cream, butter, salt and pepper, blitz until smooth and velvety, set aside
9. When the venison is soft and the sauce is nice and thick, pour it into a very large pie dish or deep-sided baking pan and spread the cauliflower mixture over the top
10. Bake in the oven at 400 degrees Fahrenheit for about 20 minutes or until the cauliflower is golden
11. Serve nice and hot!

Nutritional information:
- **Calories:** 546
- **Fat:** 36.3 grams
- **Protein:** 42.2 grams
- **Total carbs:** 11.7 grams
- **Net carbs:** 7.9 grams

Beef and Bacon Meatballs

These meatballs are golden, juicy, flavorsome and packed with keto-friendly beef and bacon. Serve them with a dipping sauce, or pile them on top of zucchini noodles with a rich bolognese sauce. The choice is yours! This is a great recipe to make with the kids as they can help to stir the mixture and roll the meatballs.

Serves: 5 (makes 15 meatballs with 3 per serving)
Time: approximately 35 minutes
Ingredients:

- 4 Tbsp olive oil for frying
- 6 rashers bacon, cut into very small pieces (or pulse them in the food processor!)
- 2 lb ground beef
- 1 egg, lightly beaten
- 1 tsp mixed dried herbs
- 1 tsp garlic powder
- Salt and pepper

Method:

1. Drizzle 1 Tbsp of the olive oil into a large, nonstick frying pan and place over a medium-high heat
2. Add the bacon to the hot pan and stir as it cooks, it should only take a couple of minutes
3. Combine the ground beef, cooked bacon, egg, herbs, garlic powder, salt and pepper in a large bowl until thoroughly combined
4. Use the same frying pan you used for the bacon and add the rest of the oil, place over a medium-high heat again
5. Roll the beef mixture into balls and fry until golden all around!
6. Serve however you wish

Note: these meatballs are great to have on hand as a super low-carb snack to grab and nibble when you've got no time to prep anything else.

Nutritional information:

- **Calories:** 484
- **Fat:** 35.4 grams
- **Protein:** 41.6 grams
- **Total carbs:** 1.1 grams
- **Net carbs:** 1 gram

Parmesan and Sunflower Seed Beef Patties

If you're a fan of burgers then you need to have a tasty keto-friendly burger pattie recipe in your repertoire, and this one is perfect! Instead of buns, just use lettuce, it adds basically NO calories and holds the burger together nice and neatly. I promise you won't even miss those carb-loaded burger buns! Serve with cheese, mayo and tomato...mouth wateringly yum.

Serves: 6 (1 large burger pattie per serving)
Time: approximately 30 minutes
Ingredients:
- 2 lb ground beef
- 2 tsp garlic powder (this stuff is amazing, make sure you buy some!)
- ¾ cup grated parmesan cheese
- 5 Tbsp sunflower seeds
- 1 egg, lightly beaten
- Salt and pepper
- Coconut or olive oil for frying

Method:
1. Combine the beef, garlic powder, parmesan, sunflower seeds, egg, salt and pepper in a large bowl until thoroughly mixed
2. Drizzle a few tablespoons of oil into a large frying pan and place over a medium-high heat
3. Roll the pattie mixture into thick patties and fry on both sides until lovely and deep golden brown
4. Assemble your keto burgers with any fillings and toppings you desire! Just remember to calculate the macros

Nutritional information:
- **Calories:** 461
- **Fat:** 33.3 grams
- **Protein:** 38.6 grams
- **Total carbs:** 2.7 grams
- **Net carbs:** 2 grams

Eggplant, Beef and Mozzarella Bake

This is the kind of dish which you simply layer into a baking dish, bake until bubbly, then serve and eat in front of a comforting movie with your family or loved one next to you. Eggplant becomes soft and gooey in the juices of the beef, and mozzarella melts to become a stringy, moreish mess.

Serves: 5
Time: approximately 45 minutes
Ingredients:
- 4 Tbsp olive oil
- 2 eggplants, thinly sliced
- ½ onion, finely chopped
- 3 tsp garlic powder
- 2 lb ground beef
- 1 cup beef stock
- 2 cups chopped spinach
- Salt and pepper
- 7 oz grated mozzarella cheese

Method:
1. Preheat the oven to 400 degrees Fahrenheit and have a baking dish standing by
2. Drizzle the olive oil into a large frying pan or saute pan and place over a medium-high heat
3. Add the eggplant slices and cook on both sides until soft, remove and set aside, keep the pan over the heat as we will use it for the beef
4. Add the onion to the pan and stir as the onion softens
5. Add the beef to the pan and stir as it becomes brown
6. Add the garlic powder, stock, spinach, salt and pepper and simmer for about 10 minutes or until the stock has reduced
7. Pour the beef mixture into your awaiting baking dish and layer the eggplant slices over top, pressing down gently to ensure they're settled snugly into the beef mixture
8. Sprinkle the mozzarella over top, place into the preheated oven and bake for about 25 minutes or until the cheese is golden and bubbly
9. Leave to cool for about 10 minutes before serving!

Nutritional information:
- **Calories:** 552
- **Fat:** 38.2 grams
- **Protein:** 46.2 grams
- **Total carbs:** 6.9 grams
- **Net carbs:** 5.7 grams

Ginger and Garlic Pork Stir Fry

Is there any dinner easier to whip together than a stir fry? Not that I can think of! This recipe features tender pork strips with fresh ginger, garlic and Asian greens. Serve with cauliflower rice, zucchini noodles, or simply on its own.

Serves: 4
Time: approximately 30 minutes
Ingredients:
- 1 Tbsp sesame oil
- 1 Tbsp peanut oil
- 1 ½ lbs pork strips
- 2 Tbsp grated fresh ginger
- 4 garlic cloves, finely chopped
- 1 tsp garlic powder
- 2 Tbsp tamari soy sauce
- 3 cups chopped bok choy
- ½ cup pork or chicken stock
- Salt and pepper
- 3 Tbsp chopped scallions
- 4 Tbsp cashews (1 Tbsp per serving)

Method:
1. Drizzle the sesame and peanut oil into a wok or large, non-stick frying pan and place over a medium-high heat
2. When the pan is nice and hot, add the pork strips and toss as they cook for a couple of minutes until brown
3. Add the ginger, garlic cloves, garlic powder and tamari and toss to combine
4. Add the bok choy to the pan, pour the stock into the pan and immediately place a lid over the pan to allow the bok choy to steam for about 1 minute
5. Take the lid off and toss everything together
6. Serve with a sprinkle of scallions and a tablespoon of cashew nuts

Nutritional information:
- **Calories:** 326
- **Fat:** 14.1 grams
- **Protein:** 39.8 grams
- **Total carbs:** 8.8 grams
- **Net carbs:** 7.5 grams

Beef Taco Cowls

Another recipe featuring the easiest meat ingredient in the world...ground beef. We cook the beef with tomatoes and spices, then pile it into a bowl with cheese, sour cream and shredded lettuce. Taco in a bowl!

Serves: 4
Time: approximately 30 minutes
Ingredients:
- 2 Tbsp olive oil
- 1 ½ lb ground beef
- 1 ½ cups tomato puree
- 2 tsp garlic powder
- 1 tsp chili powder
- 1 tsp ground paprika
- 1 tsp ground cumin
- Salt and pepper
- 3 cups shredded lettuce
- ½ red onion, finely sliced
- 4 Tbsp sour cream
- 1 cup grated cheddar cheese

Method:
1. Drizzle the olive oil into a large frying pan or sauté pan and place over a medium-high heat
2. Add the beef and stir as it becomes brown
3. Add the tomato puree, garlic powder, chili powder, paprika, cumin, salt and pepper, stir to combine and leave to simmer for about 10 minutes or until it becomes thick and rich
4. Spoon the beef mixture into four bowls and scatter with lettuce and red onion, place a dollop of sour cream on top then finish with a scattering of grated cheese
5. Serve right away, preferably with a keto margarita!

Nutritional information:
- **Calories:** 527
- **Fat:** 29.4 grams
- **Protein:** 39.9 grams
- **Total carbs:** 11.6 grams
- **Net carbs:** 9.4 grams

Rich Lamb Bolognese

This Bolognese features lamb instead of beef, for a refreshing change on a true classic. We use red wine, sun dried tomatoes, bacon, herbs and stock to create a rich, thick, earthy Bolognese sauce. Serve with zucchini noodles or simply eat alone with a grating of parmesan.

Serves: 5
Time: approximately 1 hour
Ingredients:
- 4 Tbsp olive oil
- ½ onion, finely chopped
- 2 celery sticks, finely chopped
- 6 bacon rashers, roughly chopped
- 2 lb ground lamb
- 3 tsp garlic powder
- ¼ cup sundried tomatoes, finely chopped
- 1 cup tomato puree
- ½ cup red wine
- 1 cup beef or lamb stock
- Salt and pepper
- 2 Tbsp butter

Method:
1. Drizzle the olive oil into a large sauté pan and place over a medium-high heat
2. Add the onion, celery and bacon to the hot pan and stir as the bacon sizzles and the veggies soften
3. Add the lamb and garlic powder and stir as the lamb becomes brown
4. Add the sundried tomatoes, tomato puree, wine, stock, salt and pepper and leave to simmer for 40 minutes on a low heat until reduced and thick
5. Add the butter and stir it in as it melts
6. Serve however you wish!

Note: this is a great recipe to make ahead, pack into freezer-safe containers and stash in the freezer for a later date.

Nutritional information:
- **Calories:** 588
- **Fat:** 43.2 grams
- **Protein:** 41.6 grams
- **Total carbs:** 9 grams
- **Net carbs:** 7.3 grams

Beef and Peanut Curry

If you're a little nervous about making curry, don't be! It's so easy. You just need a few spices which are handy to have in the cupboard anyway, so it's worth making the purchase. This curry is creamy and mild, with peanuts for crunch and flavor. Serve with cauliflower rice or alone with a dollop of full-fat yogurt on top.

Serves: 7 (enough for a family meal plus leftovers)
Time: approximately 1 hour
Ingredients:
- 2 Tbsp peanut oil
- ½ onion, finely chopped
- 5 garlic cloves, roughly chopped
- 3 Tbsp grated fresh ginger
- 1 fresh red chili
- 2 Tbsp ground cumin
- 1 Tbsp ground coriander seeds
- 2 Tbsp garam masala
- 2 tsp turmeric
- 1 tsp cinnamon
- Decent grind of black pepper
- 2 lbs beef cubes
- 2 Tbsp peanut butter
- ⅓ cup roasted peanuts
- 2 cups coconut cream
- Fresh cilantro

Method:
1. Drizzle the peanut oil into a large sauté pan and place over a medium heat, leave to heat up while you make the curry paste
2. Place the onion, garlic, ginger, chili, cumin, coriander, garam masala, turmeric, cinnamon and black pepper into a food processor and pulse until a thick paste forms
3. Scrape the paste into the hot pan and stir as it sizzles in the peanut oil and becomes fragrant
4. Add the beef to the pot and stir to coat in spices and become brown
5. Add the peanut butter, peanuts and coconut cream and stir to combine, leave to simmer for about 30 minutes or until thick and rich
6. Serve with a sprig of fresh cilantro on top!

Nutritional information:
- **Calories:** 565
- **Fat:** 26.8 grams
- **Protein:** 30.4 grams
- **Total carbs:** 12.2 grams
- **Net carbs:** 10 grams

Slow-Cooked Pulled Pork with Spices

Pulled pork is a wonderful thing to have stashed in the fridge to pull out for easy lunches and dinners throughout the week. Use it to fill lettuce cups, use as a base for salads or even make keto-friendly buns to make pulled pork burgers.

Serves: 8 (small servings)
Time: approximately 5 hours
Ingredients:
- Pork shoulder (about 4 pounds)
- 1 onion, roughly chopped
- 3 tsp garlic powder
- 1 Tbsp Dijon mustard
- 1 Tbsp paprika
- 1 Tbsp chili powder
- 1 Tbsp ground cumin
- 2 Tbsp Worcestershire sauce
- 2 cups chicken stock
- ⅓ cup apple cider vinegar
- Salt and pepper

Method:
1. Place all ingredients into a slow cooker and cook on high temperature for five hours
2. Lift the cooked pork out of the slow cooker and place onto a large board
3. Take two forks and shred the soft, cooked pork
4. Simmer the leftover juices and liquids to create a rich, tasty gravy to serve with the pulled pork

Nutritional information:
- **Calories:** 174
- **Fat:** 12.4 grams
- **Protein:** 12.1 grams
- **Total carbs:** 7.5 grams
- **Net carbs:** 6.5 grams

Fresh Beef Salad

One of my favorite ways to serve beef is to cook a large steak rare, slice it thinly, then toss it into a fresh, crunchy salad with a tangy dressing. An easy, fast, healthy and keto-friendly lunch or dinner.

Serves: 4
Time: approximately 25 minutes
Ingredients:
- 1 large beef rump steak, room temperature
- 2 Tbsp olive oil
- Salt and pepper
- 4 cups shredded lettuce
- 1 cup arugula
- 1 cup cucumber chunks
- 2 large tomatoes, cut into wedges or chunks
- 2 radishes, finely sliced
- 4 oz feta cheese, crumbled
- 4 Tbsp pumpkin seeds, lightly toasted on a dry frying pan

Dressing:
- 3 Tbsp olive oil
- 1 Tbsp apple cider vinegar
- Juice of 1 lemon
- 1 tsp sesame oil
- 1 tsp dried chili flakes
- Salt and pepper

Method:
1. Place a frying pan or skillet over a high heat
2. Rub the steak with olive oil, salt and pepper and place onto the hot frying pan
3. Cook the steak on both sides until dark golden on the outside and rare inside
4. Place the steak onto a board to rest while you prep the salad
5. Toss together the lettuce, arugula, cucumber, tomatoes, radishes, feta and pumpkin seeds
6. In a small cup, combine all of the dressing ingredients and pour over the salad, toss to combine
7. Slice the rested beef into thin slices and scatter over the salad before serving

Nutritional information:
- **Calories:** 473
- **Fat:** 34.3 grams
- **Protein:** 35.8 grams
- **Total carbs:** 7.7 grams
- **Net carbs:** 5.9 grams

Fish mains

Fish is such a beautiful ingredient to welcome into your weekly family menu. It contains incredibly healthy fats and lean protein to support the brain, the heart and the skin. What's more, it's fantastically keto friendly! It's best to buy fresh fish from ethical, sustainable-minded sources. For recipes featuring "fresh white fish" you can choose any white fish you like best (or can source fresh). These recipes are all extremely simple and only feature a few ingredients (mostly) so there's no need to feel overwhelmed! A few of these recipes have been created with entertaining guests in mind. Just because you're busy and you're on keto doesn't mean that your social life will stop and you'll cease to entertain friends! You'll find recipes here which are impressive and rich yet very easy and "very keto".

Pan-Seared Fresh White Fish with Butter, Lemon and Parsley

This is a fantastic recipe for keto beginners and cooking newbies. It's the best way to cook fresh fish; with a little butter, lemon and parsley on a hot frying pan.

Serves: 4
Time: approximately 20 minutes
Ingredients:
- 2 Tbsp olive oil
- 4 Tbsp butter
- 1 lb fresh white fish filets
- Juice of 1 lemon
- Salt and pepper

Method:
1. Add the olive oil and butter to a frying pan and place over a medium heat, leave to melt together until the butter is frothy
2. Add the fish to the pan and sear on both sides until deep golden on the outside and juicy on the inside
3. Squeeze the lemon juice over the fish and sprinkle with salt and pepper
4. Serve with a fresh salad!

Nutritional information:
- **Calories:** 290
- **Fat:** 19.5 grams
- **Protein:** 26.3 grams
- **Total carbs:** 0.8 grams
- **Net carbs:** 0.8 grams

Smoked Salmon and Cream Cheese Dip with Lemon Zest

Smoked salmon is a fantastic ingredient to use when you don't feel like cooking but you do want to harness the healthy fats found in salmon. Whip it with cream cheese and lemon juice and you've got yourself a retro classic. Spread onto cucumber slices or keto bagels and enjoy! You can also set this out at a dinner party with some crusty bread for non-keto dieters and veggie sticks for you and your keto companions.

Serves approximately 6
Time: approximately 10 minutes
Ingredients:
- 8 oz smoked salmon
- 10 oz plain, full-fat cream cheese
- Juice and zest of 1 lemon
- Small pinch of salt (only a tiny bit as the salmon is pretty salty already)
- Decent grind of pepper

Method:
1. Place all ingredients into a food processor and pulse until creamy
2. Spoon into a small serving bowl, cover and place into the fridge until needed

Nutritional information:
- **Calories:** 211
- **Fat:** 18.2 grams
- **Protein:** 2.5 grams
- **Total carbs:** 2.5 grams
- **Net carbs:** 2.5 grams

Oven-Baked Fish with Tomatoes and Herbs

This is a recipe which requires nothing but a tray, some fish, fresh tomatoes and a few sprigs of fresh herbs. Bake it all together, dish it up and you've got a fast, easy and comprehensive meal to impress any keto guest.

Serves: 4
Time: approximately 30 minutes
Ingredients:
- 4 fresh white fish filets (about 7 oz each)
- 2 fresh tomatoes, cut into chunks
- 1 ½ cups assorted cherry tomatoes, pricked with a fork (so they don't explode)
- 1 sprig fresh rosemary
- 1 sprig fresh thyme
- 3 Tbsp olive oil
- Salt and pepper
- 1 tsp garlic powder (my favorite as you can see!)

Method:
1. Preheat the oven to 350 degrees Fahrenheit and line a baking tray with baking paper
2. Place the fish, chopped tomatoes, cherry tomatoes and herbs onto your prepared tray and nestle them all together tightly (no need to be exact just tuck them all in)
3. Drizzle with olive oil, salt, pepper and garlic powder
4. Pop the tray into the oven and bake for about 15-20 minutes or until the fish is just cooked and the tomatoes are saucy
5. Serve right away, with sprinkle of fresh parsley!

Nutritional information:
- **Calories:** 341
- **Fat:** 13.2 grams
- **Protein:** 46.7 grams
- **Total carbs:** 4.5 grams
- **Net carbs:** 2.8 grams

Simple Fish Stir Fry with Sesame Seeds and Scallions

This dish celebrates the versatility of fish by tossing it on a hot wok with nutty sesame seeds, sweet, onion-rich scallions and a dash of tamari soy sauce. Serve alone or with keto rice or noodles.

Serves: 4
Time: approximately 20 minutes
Ingredients:
- 1 Tbsp sesame oil
- 1 Tbsp olive oil
- 1 ½ lbs fresh white fish, cut into cubes
- 2 Tbsp sesame seeds
- 3 Tbsp chopped scallions
- 2 Tbsp tamari soy sauce
- 1 tsp dried chili flakes

Method:
1. Drizzle the sesame and olive oils into a wok and place over a high heat
2. Add the fish and quickly toss as it sears
3. Add the sesame seeds, scallions, tamari and chili flakes and toss to combine everything together and allow the sesame seeds to toast
4. Serve right away to make the most of that wok heat!

Nutritional information:
- **Calories:** 285
- **Fat:** 11.6 grams
- **Protein:** 41.3 grams
- **Total carbs:** 1.9 grams
- **Net carbs:** 1.2 grams

Fish Taco Bowls

Fish tacos are the epitome of fresh, tangy goodness. However, we aren't allowed to eat taco shells on keto, so we simply leave them out. What remains is fresh, seared fish, red cabbage, sour cream, lime juice, chili and cilantro...heavenly, summery, keto-friendly and bright.

Serves: 4
Time: approximately 30 minutes
Ingredients:
- 2 Tbsp olive oil
- 1 ½ lb fresh white fish, cut into small pieces
- 1 fresh red chili, finely chopped
- Salt and pepper
- 2 cups shredded red cabbage
- 3 Tbsp chopped scallions
- 4 Tbsp sour cream
- 1 lime, quartered
- Lots of fresh cilantro, roughly chopped

Method:
1. Drizzle the olive oil into a large nonstick frying pan and place over a medium-high heat
2. Add the fish pieces, chili, salt and pepper and gently toss as the fish cooks through, take off the heat
3. In four serving bowls, divide the red cabbage and scallions, divide the fish between the bowls, add a dollop of sour cream, a lime wedge and a handful of cilantro
4. You're ready to serve!

Nutritional information:
- ***Calories:*** 305
- ***Fat:*** 12.4 grams
- ***Protein:*** 40.9 grams
- ***Total carbs:*** 6.3 grams
- ***Net carbs:*** 4.7 grams

Parmesan Crusted Fish

Instead of using carb-rich breadcrumbs to coat these fish filets, we use a mixture of parmesan cheese, herbs, garlic powder and lemon zest. The result is savory, salty and incredibly simple for anyone to make. Serve with a salad and you've created a perfect keto meal.

Serves: 4
Time: approximately 30 minutes
Ingredients:
- 3 Tbsp butter for frying
- 1 ½ lbs fresh white fish filets
- 2 Tbsp olive oil
- ¾ cups grated parmesan cheese
- Zest of 1 lemon
- 1 tsp garlic powder
- 1 tsp dried mixed herbs
- Salt and pepper

Method:
1. Place the butter into a large nonstick frying pan and place over a medium-high heat and leave to allow the butter to melt and become frothy as you prep the fish
2. On a plate, combine the parmesan, lemon zest, garlic powder, herbs, salt and pepper
3. Rub the fish with olive oil and dip both sides into the parmesan mixture before transferring directly onto the hot, buttery frying pan, fry on both sides until golden and crispy
4. Serve right away!

Note: a dollop of lemon mayo would be fabulous with this dish

Nutritional information:
- **Calories:** 408
- **Fat:** 22.9 grams
- **Protein:** 46.7 grams
- **Total carbs:** 0.8 grams
- **Net carbs:** 0.8 grams

Tuna Cakes

These little tuna cakes are filled with canned tuna (easy!), cheese, herbs and eggs to bind them together. Serve with mayo or pile into a keto burger. A yummy treat for kids and adults alike, and very easy to make for beginners.

Serves: 4
Time: approximately 30 minutes
Ingredients:
- 1 lb canned tuna, drained
- 2 eggs, lightly beaten
- 1 cup grated cheddar
- ½ cup finely chopped fresh parsley
- 4 Tbsp finely chopped scallions
- Salt and pepper
- 4 Tbsp coconut or olive oil for frying

Method:
1. Drizzle the coconut or olive oil into a nonstick frying pan and leave to heat while you prep the cakes
2. In a large bowl, combine the tuna, eggs, cheddar, parsley, scallions, salt and pepper until thoroughly combined
3. Shape the tuna mixture into little cakes or patties and fry on both sides until golden and crispy on the outside
4. Serve hot, warm or cold!

Nutritional information:
- **Calories:** 369
- **Fat:** 19.3 grams
- **Protein:** 31.8 grams
- **Total carbs:** 1.4 grams
- **Net carbs:** 1 gram

Fish with Capers, Cream, Lemon and Wine

This dish is very sophisticated and keto dinner party-worthy, but it's actually super simple. It's rich with cream and wine, with the briny flavor of capers and the tang of lemon. Best served with chilled white wine!

Serves: 4
Time: approximately 40 minutes
Ingredients:
- 2 Tbsp olive oil
- 1 lb fresh white fish filets
- 4 Tbsp capers
- ½ cup white wine
- 1 cup heavy cream
- Juice and zest of 1 lemon
- Salt and pepper
- Sprig of fresh thyme

Method:
1. Drizzle the olive oil into a large sauté pan and place over a medium-high heat
2. Add the fish to the pan and quickly sear on both sides
3. Add the capers and white wine and allow the alcohol to evaporate and the wine to come to a simmer
4. Add the cream, lemon juice and zest, salt, pepper and thyme
5. Leave to simmer on a very low heat for about 15 minutes until thick and rich
6. Serve right away, with a side salad or side of steamed asparagus

Nutritional information:
- **Calories:** 488
- **Fat:** 38 grams
- **Protein:** 28.7 grams
- **Total carbs:** 3.4 grams
- **Net carbs:** 3.1 grams

Fish and Eggplant Curry (Mild and Creamy)

Fish and eggplant are a lovely combination as they are both mild, soft and soak up flavors really well. This fish curry is mild, fragrant and tasty for even the most fearful of spices and curries.

Serves: 4
Time: approximately 45 minutes
Ingredients:
- 2 Tbsp olive oil
- 1 fresh red chili, most of the seeds removed (it reduces the spice factor), red part roughly chopped
- 3 Tbsp fresh ginger
- 4 garlic cloves
- 1 Tbsp minced lemongrass
- 1 tsp ground turmeric
- 1 tsp ground cumin
- Juice of 1 lime
- 1 ½ lbs fresh white fish, cut into cubes
- 2 eggplants, cut into cubes
- 1 cup coconut cream
- 1 cup fish stock

Method:
1. Drizzle the olive oil into a large sauté pan and place over a medium heat and leave to heat up while you make the curry paste
2. Place the chili, ginger, garlic, lemongrass, turmeric, cumin and lime juice into a food processor or blender and pulse until it forms a smooth paste
3. Add the paste to the hot pan and stir as it heats and becomes fragrant
4. Add the fish and eggplant to the pan and stir to coat in curry paste
5. Add the coconut cream and fish stock and leave to simmer for about 15 minutes
6. Serve hot, with a side of cauliflower rice!

Nutritional information:
- **Calories:** 507
- **Fat:** 31.9 grams
- **Protein:** 43.9 grams
- **Total carbs:** 10 grams
- **Net carbs:** 8 grams

Fish Skewers with Lemon Mayo

A skewer is one of the handiest, most versatile kitchen tools, and one of the most affordable too. Spike fat pieces of fresh fish onto skewers, sprinkle with spices and serve with creamy lemon mayo. Starter, lunch or snack done!

Serves: 4 (makes 8 skewers, 2 skewers per serving)
Time: approximately 30 minutes
Ingredients:
- 1 ½ lbs fresh white fish, cut into cubes
- 2 Tbsp olive oil
- 1 tsp garlic powder
- 1 tsp ground paprika
- ½ tsp chili powder
- Salt and pepper
- ½ full-fat mayo
- Juice and zest of 1 lemon
- 2 Tbsp finely chopped fresh parsley

Method:
1. Place a skillet or nonstick frying pan over a medium-high heat and leave to heat up as you prep the skewers
2. Press the fish onto the skewers but leave room at both ends for easy handling
3. Rub the fish skewers with olive oil and sprinkle with garlic powder, paprika, chili, salt and pepper
4. Place the skewers onto the hot skillet or pan and cook on all sides until golden, slightly charred, and juicy in the center
5. To make the mayo: stir together the mayo, lemon juice and zest, and parsley
6. Dip the fish skewers into the lemon mayo to serve!

Nutritional information:
- **Calories:** 464
- **Fat:** 29.7 grams
- **Protein:** 44.5 grams
- **Total carbs:** 1.6 grams
- **Net carbs:** 1.3 grams

Raw Fish Platter with Wasabi Cream

I understand if this recipe makes you a little nervous! But raw fish is one of the tastiest ways to enjoy the treats of the sea. Dip fresh salmon and tuna into wasabi mayo and tamari soy sauce and you'll see what I'm talking about. Make sure to buy the absolute freshest fish you can find, and have a very sharp knife at the ready.

Serves: 4 as a starter
Time: approximately 10 minutes
Ingredients:
- 1 fresh, raw salmon filet, skin and bones removed at the fishmonger
- 1 fresh tuna filet, skin and bones removed at the fishmonger
- 4 Tbsp Kewpie mayonnaise
- 1 tsp wasabi paste
- 4 Tbsp tamari soy sauce

Method:
1. Slice the salmon and tuna into very thin slices with a very sharp knife and layer onto a serving plate
2. Stir together the mayo and wasabi, and have the tamari soy sauce waiting in a sauce dish
3. Serve immediately to make the most of the freshness!

Nutritional information:
- **Calories:** 457
- **Fat:** 27.8 grams
- **Protein:** 43.1 grams
- **Total carbs:** 1.1 grams
- **Net carbs:** 1.1 grams

Chili Prawn Salad

Prawns are best served with a zesty salad, in my opinion. These prawns are coated in chili and tossed through a crunchy, colorful salad of red cabbage, lettuce and peanuts.

Serves: 4
Time: approximately 30 minutes
Ingredients:
- 1 lb fresh prawns, deveined
- 2 Tbsp olive oil
- 3 cups shredded red cabbage
- 2 cups shredded lettuce
- 1 ½ cups sliced cucumber
- ½ cup roasted, salted peanuts

Dressing:
- 2 Tbsp fish sauce
- 1 fresh red chili, finely chopped
- 2 Tbsp olive oil
- 1 tsp sesame oil
- Salt and pepper
- Juice of 1 lime

Method:
1. To make dressing, mix all the ingredients under dressing, put aside
2. Head a pan over medium-high heat. Add olive oil and prawns, and toss for 2 minutes or prawns change color.
3. Combine cabbage, lettuce, cucumber, salted peanuts, and prawns together, then drizzle over the dressing and toss.
4. Serve and enjoy!

Nutritional information:
- **Calories:** 373
- **Fat:** 23 grams
- **Protein:** 28.8 grams
- **Total carbs:** 12.8 grams
- **Net carbs:** 9.5 grams

Seared Scallops with Wine and Cream Sauce
(Special Occasion Recipe for Guests)

This is a recipe for when you really want to treat your guests and loved ones to something special but you don't want to attempt a very complicated recipe. Scallops are soft and decadent, and even better when cooked in wine and cream sauce. Oh, and completely keto approved!

Serves: 5
Time: approximately 30 minutes
Ingredients:
- 2 Tbsp olive oil
- 1 ½ lbs fresh scallops
- Salt and pepper
- 2 garlic cloves, finely chopped
- 2 Tbsp butter
- ½ cup dry white wine
- 1 cup heavy cream
- 1 sprig fresh thyme
- Salt and pepper

Method:
1. Place a nonstick frying pan over a medium-high heat and drizzle the olive oil into the pan
2. Place the scallops onto the hot frying pan in one layer and sear on both sides for about 2 minutes each side, sprinkle with salt and pepper then remove from the pan and set aside
3. Add the butter and garlic to the pan (it should still be on the heat) and allow the butter to melt
4. Add the wine and allow the alcohol to burn off
5. Add the cream, thyme, salt and pepper and stir to combine, allow to simmer for about 5 minutes until it starts to thicken
6. Add the scallops to the sauce and spoon the sauce over them so it covers them
7. Serve right away!

Nutritional information:
- **Calories:** 393
- **Fat:** 28.7 grams
- **Protein:** 23.9 grams
- **Total carbs:** 5.8 grams
- **Net carbs:** 5.7 grams

Prawn and Chorizo Stir Fry with Fresh Herbs and Parmesan

This may sound a little bit "off the wall" but it's actually super simple and so delicious you'll wonder where it was all your life! Chorizo gives a smoky, salty flavor to the soft prawns, with parmesan adding more saltiness and creaminess, with fresh herbs adding color and life.

Serves: 4
Time: approximately 30 minutes
Ingredients:
- 2 Tbsp olive oil
- 5 oz chorizo sausage, cut into disks
- 1 ½ lb prawns, deveined
- ½ cup chopped fresh parsley
- ¼ cup chopped fresh cilantro
- ½ cup grated parmesan cheese

To serve:
- 3 Tbsp olive oil
- Juice of 1 lemon

Method:
1. Drizzle the first measure of olive oil into a frying pan or skillet and place over a medium-high heat
2. Add the chorizo to the pan and fry until each side becomes golden and the oils melt out of the sausage and into the pan
3. Add the prawns to the pan and cook until they turn pink and cooked through, remove from the heat
4. Add the parsley, cilantro, parmesan, olive oil and lemon juice to the chorizo and prawns and toss to gently combine
5. Serve!

Nutritional information:
- **Calories:** 447
- **Fat:** 29.1 grams
- **Protein:** 46.3 grams
- **Total carbs:** 3.3 grams
- **Net carbs:** 2 grams

Chicken Dishes

We've reached the chicken section! Chicken is a favorite for a reason. It's versatile, healthy, easy to prepare and goes with absolutely any flavor you throw at it. Chicken is a true keto champion ingredient as it's super low carb, provides healthy protein and can be enjoyed for lunch or dinner. These recipes are all incredibly simple and fast for you to prepare easily, even when you're not in the mood for cooking.

Oven-Baked Drumsticks with Sesame Seeds

Starting off with the easiest chicken dish ever, oven-baked drumsticks! These drumsticks are flavored with nutty sesame oil, sesame seeds and soy sauce. Nibble them for lunch with a salad, or eat as a mid-morning snack.

Serves: 4 (2 drumsticks each)
Time: approximately 30 minutes
Ingredients:
- 8 chicken drumsticks
- 3 Tbsp olive oil
- 2 tsp sesame oil
- 3 Tbsp tamari soy sauce
- 4 Tbsp sesame seeds
- Salt and pepper

Method:
1. Preheat the oven to 400 degrees Fahrenheit and line a baking tray with baking paper
2. Place the drumsticks onto the tray and drizzle over the olive oil, sesame oil, tamari, sesame seeds, salt and pepper
3. Use your hands to rub the oils and seeds into the drumsticks to they are all evenly coated
4. Pop the tray into the oven and bake for about 25 minutes or until cooked through
5. Eat hot, warm or cold!

Nutritional information:
- **Calories:** 530
- **Fat:** 36.8 grams
- **Protein:** 47 grams
- **Total carbs:** 2.9 grams
- **Net carbs:** 1.8 grams

Chicken Thighs with Sun Dried Tomato Cream Sauce

Chicken thighs pan fried in olive oil, then doused in a creamy sauce made from wine, sun dried tomatoes and cream. Incredibly rich and tasty! You could absolutely whip this dish together to impress your guests without going to too much trouble.

Serves: 4
Time: approximately 35 minutes
Ingredients:
- 3 Tbsp olive oil
- 4 large boneless chicken thighs
- Salt and pepper
- 4 garlic cloves, finely chopped
- ½ cup wine
- ⅓ cup finely chopped sun-dried tomatoes
- 2 Tbsp tomato paste
- 1 cup heavy cream

Method:
1. Drizzle the olive oil into a sauté pan and place over a medium-high heat
2. Add the chicken thighs to the hot pan and sprinkle both sides with salt and pepper, cook on both sides until golden and almost cooked right through
3. Add the garlic and wine to the pan and allow the alcohol to burn off the wine, about 2 minutes
4. Add the sun-dried tomatoes, tomato paste and cream, and stir to combine, allow to simmer for about 10 minutes
5. Serve with a sprinkle of fresh herbs and a side salad!

Nutritional information:
- **Calories:** 543
- **Fat:** 46.2 grams
- **Protein:** 19.6 grams
- **Total carbs:** 10 grams
- **Net carbs:** 8.2 grams

Chicken Stir Fry with Orange and Scallions

Chicken breast strips stir fried with orange zest, orange juice and scallions. Serve alone or with cauliflower rice! Light, fresh, different and satisfying.

Serves: 4
Time: approximately 30 minutes
Ingredients:
- 2 Tbsp olive oil
- 2 Tbsp butter
- 2 large chicken breasts, skinless, cut into strips
- Zest and juice of 1 orange
- 4 Tbsp finely chopped scallions
- Salt and pepper

Method:
1. Place the olive oil and butter into a nonstick frying pan and place over a medium-high heat
2. Add the chicken breast pieces to the hot pan and stir as they cook until almost cooked through
3. Add the orange zest, juice, scallions, salt and pepper and stir to combine
4. Allow to cook for another couple of minutes to allow the chicken to cook through
5. Serve hot!

Nutritional information:
- **Calories:** 259
- **Fat:** 13.6 grams
- **Protein:** 29 grams
- **Total carbs:** 2.7 grams
- **Net carbs:** 2.4 grams

Chicken and Mozzarella Patties

These patties can be used for burgers or eaten alone with a variety of keto dipping sauces as a quick snack or easy starter. Ground chicken is a light and tasty change from ground beef, and it goes deliciously well with oozing mozzarella.

Serves: 4 (makes 16 patties with 4 patties per serving)
Time: approximately 30 minutes
Ingredients:
- 2 lbs ground chicken
- 2 tsp garlic powder
- 1 egg, lightly beaten
- 1 ½ cups grated mozzarella
- ½ cup finely chopped parsley
- Salt and pepper
- 4 Tbsp oil for frying

Method:
1. In a large bowl, combine the chicken, garlic powder, egg, mozzarella, parsley, salt and pepper
2. Drizzle the olive oil into a large nonstick frying pan and place over a medium-high heat
3. Shape the chicken mixture into patties and place into the hot frying pan, cook on both sides until golden and cooked right through
4. Serve however you wish!

Nutritional information:
- **Calories:** 611
- **Fat:** 45.3 grams
- **Protein:** 49.7 grams
- **Total carbs:** 3.2 grams
- **Net carbs:** 2.8 grams

Chicken, Broccoli and Cashew Stir Fry

An easy stir fry with chicken breast, crunchy broccoli and salty cashews. The epitome of a perfect weeknight keto dinner. You get protein, healthy fats and leafy green veggies packed with nutrients...all in one easy dish.

Serves: 4
Time: 30 minutes
Ingredients:
- 3 Tbsp olive oil
- 2 large chicken breasts, skinless, sliced into small pieces
- 1 tsp garlic powder
- 4 cups broccoli florets
- ¼ cup roasted, salted cashew nuts
- 3 Tbsp tamari soy sauce
- Salt and pepper

Method:
1. Drizzle the olive oil into a wok and place over a high heat
2. Add the chicken and toss as it cooks and becomes golden
3. Add the garlic powder, broccoli, cashews, soy sauce, salt and pepper and stir as the broccoli cooks slightly but still remains crunchy
4. Serve super hot!

Nutritional information:
- **Calories:** 316
- **Fat:** 15.2 grams
- **Protein:** 34.7 grams
- **Total carbs:** 10.1 grams
- **Net carbs:** 7.5 grams

Whole Roasted Chicken with Roasted Cauliflower

Excellent

Here we have a roast chicken! A simple classic you can tear apart and eat for lunch and dinner in a variety of ways. We use butter, lemon and herbs to flavor the chicken, and tuck cauliflower around the chicken to roast in the chicken juices.

Serves 6
Time: approximately 1 hour 20 minutes
Ingredients:
- 1 large whole chicken
- 2 Tbsp butter, soft
- 3 Tbsp olive oil
- Salt and pepper
- 1 lemon
- 1 sprig fresh rosemary
- 1 sprig fresh thyme
- 3 cups cauliflower florets
- 2 tsp garlic powder

Method:
1. Preheat the oven to 400 degrees Fahrenheit and have a roasting dish standing by
2. Place the chicken into the roasting pan and rub the soft butter and olive oil over the top
3. Place the lemon and herbs into the cavity of the chicken
4. Tuck the cauliflower florets around the chicken, drizzle them with a little more olive oil and sprinkle with garlic powder, salt and pepper
5. Slip the pan into the oven and roast for about an hour and 10 minutes or until the chicken is cooked all the way through (check by cutting down to the bone next to the thigh joint to see if it's fully cooked)
6. Leave to rest for 10 minutes before carving and devouring!

Nutritional information:
- **Calories:** 308
- **Fat:** 19.3 grams
- **Protein:** 28.2 grams
- **Total carbs:** 4.7 grams
- **Net carbs:** 3.3 grams

Chicken Wings with Chili-Lime Aioli

Chicken wings are a crowd pleaser whether you're entertaining or simply whipping something up to feed the family as a tasty snack. We serve these ones with aioli mixed with chili and lime for heat and zest.

Serves: 4
Time: approximately 30 minutes
Ingredients:
- 2 lb chicken wings
- 3 Tbsp olive oil
- 2 Tbsp hot chili sauce
- 2 tsp garlic powder
- Salt and pepper
- ½ cup full-fat aioli
- ½ fresh red chili, finely chopped
- Juice of 1 lime

Method:
1. Preheat the oven to 400 degrees Fahrenheit and line a baking tray with baking paper
2. Spread the wings onto the tray and drizzle over the olive oil, hot sauce, garlic powder, salt and pepper. Use your hands to massage everything into the wings
3. Slip the tray into the oven and bake for about 25 minutes or until the wings are cooked through (each oven is different, so be sure to check)
4. Mix together the aioli, red chili and lime juice in a serving bowl
5. Serve the wings nice and hot!

Nutritional information:
- **Calories:** 545
- **Fat:** 46.3 grams
- **Protein:** 28.4 grams
- **Total carbs:** 2.5 grams
- **Net carbs:** 2.3 grams

Chicken, Mushroom and Leek Stew

This is the kind of stew the whole family can enjoy. Tender chicken swims in creamy mushroom and leek gravy after being slow cooked for four hours. Highly recommended for colder seasons!

Serves: 5
Time: approximately 4 and a half hours
Ingredients:
- 3 Tbsp olive oil
- ½ onion, finely chopped
- 1 ½ lb chicken thighs, boneless
- 3 cups sliced mushrooms
- 1 cup sliced leeks
- 2 tsp garlic powder
- 2 cups chicken stock
- 1 cup heavy cream
- 1 tsp arrowroot powder dissolved in 2 tsp water
- Salt and pepper

Method:
1. Drizzle the olive oil into a large, oven-safe pot and place over a medium-high heat
2. Add the onion and chicken and stir to brown the chicken and soften the onions
3. Add the mushrooms and leeks and stir as they soften together
4. Add the garlic powder, stock, cream, arrowroot mixture, salt and pepper and stir to combine
5. Bring to a boil before reducing to a gentle simmer over a low heat and allow to simmer for four hours
6. Serve steaming hot

Nutritional information:
- **Calories:** 500
- **Fat:** 38.2 grams
- **Protein:** 29.1 grams
- **Total carbs:** 10 grams
- **Net carbs:** 8.7 grams

Chicken, Feta and Olive Salad

A fresh salad with herbed chicken breast, salty feta cheese and briny olives. It's reminiscent of a classic Greek salad, and it's filling as well as refreshing.

Serves: 4
Time: approximately 30 minutes
Ingredients:
- 2 large chicken breasts, skinless
- 2 Tbsp olive oil
- 2 tsp dried mixed herbs
- Salt and pepper
- 6 cups shredded lettuce
- 20 black olives, pitted
- 5 oz feta cheese, crumbled
- 2 large tomatoes, cut into wedges
- ⅓ red onion, sliced
- 3 Tbsp olive oil
- Juice of 1 lemon

Method:
1. Preheat the oven to 400 degrees Fahrenheit and line a baking tray with baking paper
2. Place the chicken breasts onto the tray and rub with olive oil, herbs, salt and pepper
3. Pop the tray into the oven and cook the chicken for about 20 minutes or until cooked right through
4. Leave the chicken to rest as you prep the salad
5. In a large salad bowl, toss the lettuce, olives, feta, tomatoes, red onion, olive oil and lemon juice
6. Slice the chicken and scatter over the salad right before serving

Nutritional information:
- **Calories:** 453
- **Fat:** 29.5 grams
- **Protein:** 36.4 grams
- **Total carbs:** 6.1 grams
- **Net carbs:** 4.7 grams

Slow-Cooked Chicken Chili

Imagine a steaming bowl of rich, spicy chicken chili on a freezing Winter night. Topped with sour cream, scallions and cheese (just a suggestion, it's all up to you!). Mmmm, yum. That's what we've got for you here! Easy, slow-cooked chicken chili...warm and rich in flavor.

Serves: 5
Time: approximately 6 hours
Ingredients:
- 2 Tbsp olive oil
- 2 lb ground chicken
- ½ onion, finely chopped
- 2 cups tomato puree
- 1 Tbsp garlic powder
- 1 Tbsp paprika
- 1 Tbsp chili powder
- Salt and pepper

Method:
1. Place all ingredients into your slow cooker, pop the lid on, set the temperature to low and set the time to 6 hours
2. When the time is up, give the chili a good stir and taste it. If it needs more seasoning or flavor, add it!
3. Serve piping hot

Nutritional information:
- **Calories:** 386
- **Fat:** 23.6 grams
- **Protein:** 34.8 grams
- **Total carbs:** 11.7 grams
- **Net carbs:** 9.6 grams

Chicken and Tomato Tray Bake

Here we have another tray bake! An oven and a tray is all you need to cook a wholesome, well-rounded keto meal, and this one features chicken, tomatoes, peppers and a little cheeky hit of cream cheese.

Serves: 5
Time: approximately 40 minutes
Ingredients:
- 7 chicken thighs, boneless
- 3 large tomatoes, cut into chunks
- 1 cup cherry tomatoes, pricked with a knife or fork
- 2 red bell peppers, core and seeds removed, sliced
- 2 tsp garlic powder
- 4 Tbsp olive oil
- Salt and pepper
- 5 Tbsp cream cheese

Method:
1. Preheat the oven to 400 degrees Fahrenheit and line a baking tray with baking paper
2. Place the chicken thighs, tomato chunks, cherry tomatoes and red pepper slices onto the tray and nestle them together
3. Sprinkle the garlic powder, olive oil, salt and pepper over the chicken and veggies and use your hands to rub everything together
4. Break up the cream cheese into small pieces and dot them over the chicken and veggies
5. Slip the tray into the oven and bake for about 25 minutes or until the chicken is cooked through
6. Serve!

Nutritional information:
- **Calories:** 434
- **Fat:** 32.7 grams
- **Protein:** 24.6 grams
- **Total carbs:** 9.2 grams
- **Net carbs:** 6.6 grams

Chicken and Bell Pepper Fajitas

Friday night should always be fajita night! These fajitas are made with sizzling chicken, charred bell peppers, cheese and sour cream. We can't accompany these with tortilla chips or taco shells (not keto friendly!) but honestly, you won't even miss them as this dish is filling enough as it is.

Serves: 4
Time: approximately 30 minutes
Ingredients:
- 2 large chicken breasts, skinless, sliced into thin slices
- 2 green bell peppers, thinly sliced
- 4 Tbsp olive oil
- 1 Tbsp paprika
- 1 Tbsp chili powder
- 1 Tbsp garlic powder
- 1 cup grated cheddar
- ½ cup sour cream
- 1 lime, quartered

Method:
1. Place a skillet over a high heat and drizzle with olive oil
2. Add the chicken and peppers to the hot skillet and sprinkle over the paprika, chili powder and garlic powder
3. Stir as the chicken and peppers cook through and become soft and charred, take off the heat
4. Pile the chicken and peppers onto a serving plate and put the cheese and sour cream into their own serving bowls for your guests to help themselves, each with a lime quarter for a drizzle of sourness

Nutritional information:
- **Calories:** 452
- **Fat:** 22.2 grams
- **Protein:** 33.6 grams
- **Total carbs:** 10 grams
- **Net carbs:** 7.3 grams

Chicken and Avocado Sushi

I couldn't possibly get to the end of this section without including a little sushi treat. Chicken breast, creamy avocado and even creamier cream cheese all rolled into a nori sheet and sprinkled with sesame seeds.

Serves: 4
Time: approximately 35 minutes
Ingredients:
- 1 large chicken breast, cut into small pieces
- 2 Tbsp olive oil
- 2 Tbsp tamari soy sauce
- Salt and pepper
- 4 nori sheets
- 1 avocado, flesh sliced
- 4 Tbsp cream cheese, softened
- 4 Tbsp toasted sesame seeds

Method:
1. Place a non-stick frying pan over a medium-high heat and drizzle the olive oil into the pan
2. Add the chicken, tamari, salt and pepper and stir as the chicken cooks all the way through, set aside
3. Lay a nori sheet onto a sushi mat and spread a stripe of cream cheese through the center, horizontally. Lay a few avocado slices and chicken pieces over the cream cheese and sprinkle the sesame seeds over the top
4. Carefully roll the sushi and seal the edges with a little water on your finger
5. Slice and serve!

Nutritional information:
- **Calories:** 274
- **Fat:** 19.3 grams
- **Protein:** 19.2 grams
- **Total carbs:** 7.6 grams
- **Net carbs:** 3 grams

Loaded Keto Smoothies

We have a dedicated smoothie section here because smoothies are FANTASTIC on a beginner's keto diet (I know there are a couple of smoothies up there in the breakfast section, but we need more, more, MORE!). Smoothies are so easy to make. You can pack them full of all the macronutrients you need and simply sip on the go for breakfast, lunch or a snack. Instead of using the usual smoothie staple, the banana, we use avocado instead. Avocados give the smooth, creamy texture of a traditional smoothie, but with fewer carbs, more fiber and LOTS of healthy fats. We also use fat sources such as chia seeds, olive oil and flaxseeds. It's worth buying a carton or two of unsweetened almond milk because that's the liquid base for most of these smoothies. Just remember to check the macros on the bottle to make sure you're buying a low-carb variety.

Avocado and Strawberry Smoothie

This smoothie combines the green goodness of avocado with the rich, red, vitamin-C goodness of strawberries. We add spinach for extra nutrients and olive oil for velvety smoothness and keto-loving fats.

Serves: 2
Time: 5 minutes
Ingredients:
- 1 avocado
- ½ cup sliced strawberries
- 1 cup spinach leaves
- 1 cup of ice
- 10 almonds
- 2 Tbsp olive oil
- 1 ½ cups almond milk

Method:
1. Pop all ingredients into your blender and blend until you reach a creamy, smooth consistency
2. Serve right away

Nutritional information:
- **Calories:** 299
- **Fat:** 27.7 grams
- **Protein:** 3.7 grams
- **Total carbs:** 11.5 grams
- **Net carbs:** 3.8 grams

Cinnamon Bun Smoothie

This smoothie evokes the warming deliciousness of cinnamon buns. We use stevia to sweeten the deal and almond butter for fats, vitamin E and extra thickness.

Serves: 2
Time: 5 minutes
Ingredients:
- 1 avocado
- 2 tsp cinnamon
- 1 tsp stevia
- 2 Tbsp almond butter
- Handful of ice
- 1 ½ cups almond milk

Method:
1. Blend all the ingredients together in your blender until velvety
2. Pour into tall glasses and serve immediately

Note: an extra sprinkle of cinnamon on top would be tasty and stylish!

Nutritional information:
- **Calories:** 251
- **Fat:** 21.4 grams
- **Protein:** 5.8 grams
- **Total carbs:** 11.8 grams
- **Net carbs:** 2.7 grams

Super Green Smoothie

Green smoothies power your morning with nutrients provided by fresh veggies and fats. This is a great smoothie to choose when you feel like you just need an extra dose of health, perhaps after an indulgent weekend?

Serves: 2
Time: 5 minutes
Ingredients:
- 1 avocado
- 1 cup spinach
- ½ cup cucumber
- ½ cup celery
- Juice of 1 lime
- ⅓ green apple
- 2 Tbsp olive oil
- 1 cup of ice
- 2 cups almond milk

Method:
1. Throw everything into a large blender jug and blend until smooth. It might take a few extra pulses to get any grittiness or chunkiness out of the apple and celery
2. Pour and serve ASAP

Nutritional information:
- **Calories:** 298
- **Fat:** 26.7 grams
- **Protein:** 3.4 grams
- **Total carbs:** 15 grams
- **Net carbs:** 7.3 grams

Chocolate Raspberry Smoothie

This smoothie contains cocoa powder which is filled with antioxidants...plus, it gives this smoothie a delectable chocolate flavor! Raspberries are nutritious, tangy and sweet, with coconut oil adding delicious fat to get our macros in place.

Serves: 2
Time: 5 minutes
Ingredients:
- 1 avocado
- 2 Tbsp unsweetened cocoa powder
- ½ tsp stevia
- ½ cup raspberries
- 2 Tbsp coconut oil
- 1 cup of ice
- 1 ½ cups almond milk

Method:
1. Add everything to your blender and blend until smooth and creamy
2. Serve immediately!

Tip: A dusting of cocoa on top would be lovely

Nutritional information:
- **Calories:** 295
- **Fat:** 27.1 grams
- **Protein:** 3.6 grams
- **Total carbs:** 13.4 grams
- **Net carbs:** 3.7 grams

Peanut Butter and Jam Smoothie

This smoothie combines peanut butter with strawberries to create that beloved flavor combination...PB & J! We add a little cream to the mix for extra fat macros. This smoothie is great for days when you feel like something a wee bit sweet and naughty.

Serves: 2
Time: 5 minutes
Ingredients:
- 1 avocado
- 2 Tbsp peanut butter
- ½ cup strawberry halves
- ½ tsp stevia
- 2 Tbsp coconut oil
- ½ cup heavy cream
- 1 cup almond milk
- ½ cup ice

Method:
1. Add all ingredients to your blender and blend until super smooth and creamy
2. Pour into tall glasses and serve with a little sliver of strawberry on the side of the glass

Nutritional information:
- **Calories:** 568
- **Fat:** 55.9 grams
- **Protein:** 6.9 grams
- **Total carbs:** 15.4 grams
- **Net carbs:** 8 grams

Wake-Me-Up Coffee Smoothie

Can you start your day properly without a hit of coffee? Me neither. This smoothie combines delicious coffee with filling and nutritious avocado, coconut oil, walnuts and almond milk.

Serves: 2
Time: 5 minutes
Ingredients:
- 3 tsp instant espresso powder, mixed with 2 Tbsp hot water water (just mix it right in your blender)
- 1 avocado
- 2 Tbsp coconut oil
- 3 Tbsp walnuts
- ½ tsp stevia
- 1 cup of ice
- ⅓ cup heavy cream
- 1 cup almond milk

Method:
1. Toss everything into your blender and blitz until velvety smooth
2. Consume right away!

Nutritional information:
- **Calories:** 429
- **Fat:** 44.2 grams
- **Protein:** 3.5 grams
- **Total carbs:** 8.6 grams
- **Net carbs:** 2.7 grams

Berries and Cream Smoothie

A traditional flavor combo: berries and cream, like a sweet Summer dessert! Only this version is much healthier and totally keto friendly. Use fresh or frozen berries, whatever you can source!

Serves: 2
Time: 5 minutes
Ingredients:
- ⅓ cup strawberry halves
- ⅓ cup raspberries
- ⅓ cup boysenberries
- ½ cup heavy cream
- ½ tsp stevia
- 1 avocado
- 2 Tbsp olive oil
- 1 cup ice
- 1 cup almond milk

Method:
1. Pop everything into your blender jug and blend until creamy
2. Devour right now!

Nutritional information:
- **Calories:** 491
- **Fat:** 48.1 grams
- **Protein:** 3.8 grams
- **Total carbs:** 15.5 grams
- **Net carbs:** 7 grams

Mint Choc Chip Smoothie

Mmmmm, mint choc chip...the best ice cream flavor ever? Controversial, I know. This smoothie is inspired by mint choc chip ice cream, featuring fresh mint leaves and unsweetened cocoa powder.

Serves: 2
Time: 5 minutes
Ingredients:
- 1 avocado
- ⅓ cup fresh mint leaves
- 2 Tbsp unsweetened cocoa powder
- ½ tsp stevia
- 1 cup spinach
- 2 Tbsp almond butter
- 1 cup ice
- 1 ½ cups almond milk

Method:
1. You know the drill, load all of the ingredients into your blender and blitz, blitz, blitz until creamy
2. Serve immediately and enjoy

Nutritional information:
- **Calories:** 270
- **Fat:** 22.2 grams
- **Protein:** 7.2 grams
- **Total carbs:** 15.9 grams
- **Net carbs:** 5.8 grams

Mango, Spinach and Strawberry Smoothie

This smoothie has a little tropical touch to it with the addition of mango. We don't use a lot, as too much mango can push the carb count overboard, but just a small amount is enough to achieve amazing sweetness and deep flavor. We add spinach for nutrients and strawberries for sweetness and vitamin C.

Serves: 2
Time: 5 minutes
Ingredients:
- ½ cup mango flesh
- 1 cup spinach
- ½ cup sliced strawberries
- 2 Tbsp olive oil
- 1 cup ice
- 1 avocado
- 1 ½ cups almond milk

Method:
1. Pack all of the ingredients into your blender and blitz until smooth and creamy
2. Serve right away and enjoy

Nutritional information:
- **Calories:** 299
- **Fat:** 26.2 grams
- **Protein:** 3.2 grams
- **Total carbs:** 16.4 grams
- **Net carbs:** 8.9 grams

Creamy Chia and Vanilla Smoothie

Chia seeds provide amazing fiber as well as absolutely beautiful, healthy fats. We add vanilla for that warm, comforting flavor and cream for a hit of, well...creaminess! We hydrate the chia seeds for 10 minutes before adding them to the blender, so bear that in mind when planning.

Serves: 2
Time: 15 minutes (including 10 minutes to hydrate the chia seeds)
Ingredients:
- 3 Tbsp chia seeds hydrated in 6 Tbsp water for 10 minutes
- 1 ½ Tbsp pure vanilla extract
- 1 avocado
- ½ cup heavy cream
- 1 cup almond milk
- 1 cup of ice

Method:
1. Pop everything into the blender (including the hydrated chia seeds) and blend until velvety
2. Serve immediately

Nutritional information:
- **Calories:** 452
- **Fat:** 38.3 grams
- **Protein:** 7.6 grams
- **Total carbs:** 16.8 grams
- **Net carbs:** 3.8 grams

Coconut and Lime Smoothie

Another smoothie inspired by the tropics. This one kind of feels like you're sipping on a creamy cocktail, only far healthier. We combine lime juice and zest, coconut cream, avocado and cashews to create a fat-rich smoothie with a heavenly flavor profile.

Serves: 2
Time: 5 minutes
Ingredients:
- Zest and juice of 2 limes
- 1 avocado
- ¾ cup full-fat coconut cream
- 1 cup almond milk
- ½ tsp stevia
- 3 Tbsp raw cashews
- 1 cup of ice

Method:
1. Add everything to your blender and blitz until absolutely and totally creamy and smooth
2. Serve and sip right away

Nutritional information:
- **Calories:** 355
- **Fat:** 32 grams
- **Protein:** 5.9 grams
- **Total carbs:** 14.6 grams
- **Net carbs:** 8 grams

Blueberry and Almond Butter Smoothie

Blueberries are known for their incredibly high levels of antioxidants, so of course we want to make the most of them. We combine these sweet, bold little berries with almond butter for texture and fat, with a little hint of vanilla for extra flavor depth and of course, an avocado and a pour of almond milk.

Serves: 2
Time: 5 minutes
Ingredients:
- ¾ cup blueberries
- 1 avocado
- 2 Tbsp almond butter
- 1 tsp pure vanilla extract
- 1 cup of ice
- 1 ½ cups almond milk

Method:
1. Add all ingredients into your blender and blend until the texture is lovely and smooth
2. Serve and sip

Nutritional information:
- **Calories:** 266
- **Fat:** 21.5 grams
- **Protein:** 6 grams
- **Total carbs:** 15 grams
- **Net carbs:** 6.4 grams

Halloween Pumpkin Spice Smoothie

This smoothie is inspired by the ever-popular Halloween flavor combination...pumpkin spice! You do need to cook some pumpkin for this recipe, which does increase the time, but you could also use leftover pumpkin from dinner if you happen to have some! We don't use a lot of pumpkin, as too much can increase the carb count too much, but yes, pumpkin is allowed on keto!

Serves: 2

Time: 5 minutes (plus time to cook the pumpkin if you're cooking it from scratch. Just pop it in a steamer over a pot of boiling water and steam until super soft)

Ingredients:
- ¾ cup cooked pumpkin
- 1 tsp cinnamon
- ½ tsp allspice
- ½ tsp ground ginger
- ½ tsp stevia
- 1 avocado
- 2 Tbsp coconut oil
- 1 cup of ice
- 1 ½ cups almond milk

Method:
1. Load all ingredients into your blender and blitz until totally smooth and thick
2. Pour and sip with a straw a spare moment to yourself

Nutritional information:

Calories: 286
Fat: 26.9 grams
Protein: 3 grams
Total carbs: 14 grams
Net carbs: 5.4 grams

Sweet Treats, Desserts and Sweet Drinks

Just because baked goods and sugary foods are out of bounds, we can still enjoy sweet treats when on the keto diet. We can enjoy berries, cocoa, cream, peanut butter...and so many other goodies. And of course, we have stevia to help us achieve that sweetness we crave. This section includes little morsels such as truffles and fat bombs, and simple desserts such as berries and cream. But we also include sweet drinks such as hot chocolate and chai latte. These recipes are all super easy and fast to whip together because I know you don't have the time to muck around in the kitchen for hours!

Just a note on stevia: start with the recommended amount in the ingredients list but always taste the dish to see if it's sweet enough. If not? Add a touch more. Or, if you prefer a very, very subtle sweetness, you could always add less stevia than what's recommended then add more as needed.

Chocolate Truffles

These chocolate truffles contain only 3 ingredients, including dark chocolate. Remember to buy dark chocolate with a cocoa content of at least 72% to make sure it's keto friendly.

Serves: 20 (1 truffle per serving)

Time: 15 minutes prep time plus 1 hour in the fridge

Ingredients:
- 8 oz 72% cocoa dark chocolate
- 1 cup heavy cream
- 2 Tbsp coconut oil

Method:
1. Place the chocolate, cream and coconut oil into a glass bowl and place it over a saucepan of boiling water on the stove and gently melt, stirring every once in a while
2. Place the bowl into the fridge to set for an hour
3. Prepare a tray by lining with baking paper
4. Take a spoon and roll the mixture into balls and set them onto your lined baking tray
5. Pop them back into the fridge until needed
6. Once they're entirely set, you can store them in an airtight container

Nutritional information:
- **Calories:** 109
- **Fat:** 9.7 grams
- **Protein:** 1.5 grams
- **Total carbs:** 6.2 grams
- **Net carbs:** 6.2 grams

Peanut Butter Fat Bombs

These little round bombs are filled with peanut butter, cream, stevia and ground almonds. They're perfect for anyone who loves the combination of sweet and salty.

Serves: 15 (1 fat bomb per serving)
Time: 15 minutes prep time plus overnight to set in the fridge
Ingredients:
- 1 cup organic (no additives) peanut butter, smooth or crunchy
- 1 tsp stevia
- 1 cup heavy cream
- ½ cup ground almonds
- Pinch of sea salt

Method:
1. Line a baking tray with baking paper
2. Place the peanut butter, stevia and cream into a microwave-safe bowl and blast in the microwave for about 10 seconds, just to soften the peanut butter enough to stir properly
3. Add the ground almonds and salt and stir thoroughly to combine
4. Roll the mixture into balls and place them onto your prepared baking tray and pop into the fridge overnight
5. Pack away into an airtight container and enjoy!

Nutritional information:
- **Calories:** 175
- **Fat:** 16 grams
- **Protein:** 4.7 grams
- **Total carbs:** 5.4 grams
- **Net carbs:** 4 grams

Berries and Cream Pots

This dessert is just as it sounds, fresh berries with sweet, pillowy whipped cream all piled into dessert dishes and sprinkled with a little cocoa just for color and a shadow of chocolate flavor.

Serves: 4
Time: 10 minutes
Ingredients:
- ½ cup sliced strawberries
- ½ cup raspberries
- ½ cup blueberries
- 1 ½ cup heavy cream
- ½ tsp stevia
- 1 tsp pure vanilla
- Dusting of cocoa powder

Method:
1. Place the cream, stevia and vanilla into a bowl and whip until soft and thick but not stiff
2. Stir the berries into the sweetened cream and spoon into four dessert dishes
3. Store in the fridge until needed
4. Before serving, dust with a little cocoa powder

Nutritional information:
Calories: 338
Fat: 33.3 grams
Protein: 2.2 grams
Total carbs: 8.9 grams
Net carbs: 7 grams

Coconut Berry Ice Cream

YES you can make keto ice cream! All you need is a pile of frozen berries, coconut cream, a hit of stevia and voila. Oh, and you also need a little patience to wait for it to set properly, but you can walk away and live life as you do so.

Serves: 8
Time: about 10 minutes prep time plus about 4 hours in the freezer
Ingredients:

- 1 cup frozen raspberries
- 1 cup frozen strawberries
- 1 cup frozen boysenberries
- Juice of 1 lemon
- 1 cup full-fat coconut cream
- 1 cup heavy cream
- 1 tsp stevia

Method:

1. Place all ingredients into your food processor and blend until smooth, thick and creamy
2. Spoon into an empty ice cream container or airtight container and pop into the freezer
3. Give the ice cream a stir every half an hour or so (if you're home and you can be bothered)
4. Scoop into little bowls or cups and enjoy with a little spoon!

Nutritional information:
Calories: 178
Fat: 16.3 grams
Protein: 1.6 grams
Total carbs: 7.4 grams
Net carbs: 5.1 grams

Vanilla Choc Chip Ice Cream

Another ice cream recipe! This one is a combination of two classics: vanilla and chocolate chips. Remember to use 100% pure vanilla extract and not vanilla imitation or essence.

Serves: 10

Time: 1 hour to prep (including cooling time so only about 10 minutes of active cooking time) and about 4 hours to freeze

Ingredients:
- 2 cups heavy cream
- 3 egg yolks
- 2 Tbsp pure vanilla extract
- 1 tsp stevia
- 1 cup finely chopped 72% cocoa dark chocolate

Method:
1. Place the cream, egg yolks, vanilla and stevia into a large bowl and place over a saucepan of boiling water
2. Whisk to combine and keep whisking as the mixture slightly thickens
3. Take the bowl off the heat and leave to cool
4. Stir the chocolate into the cream mixture and pour into an empty ice cream container or airtight container
5. Pop into the fridge and stir every half hour if you can
6. Give the ice cream a good, hard stir before scooping and serving

Nutritional information:
- *Calories:* 246
- *Fat:* 22.9 grams
- *Protein:* 3 grams
- *Total carbs:* 7.8 grams
- *Net carbs:* 7.8 grams

Almond and Peanut Butter Chocolate Cookie Bites

These aren't what you would usually think of as a cookie. They're in the shape of a cookie, but the texture is more similar to fudge. We use almond butter AND peanut butter, and cover it with melted chocolate. I guess it's kind of like a Reese's cup but with almonds added...and minus all the sugar.

Serves: 20 (1 cookie bite per serving)
Time: 30 minutes prep time plus about 3 hours to set
Ingredients:
- ¾ cup organic (no additives) peanut butter, smooth or crunchy
- ¾ cup almond butter
- Pinch of salt
- ½ tsp stevia
- 5 oz 72% cocoa dark chocolate

Method:
1. Line a baking tray with baking paper
2. In a large bowl, combine the peanut butter, almond butter, salt and stevia
3. Roll spoonfuls of nut butter mixture into balls and then press them into cookie shapes on your prepared tray
4. Place the tray into the fridge to allow the cookies to set while you melt the chocolate
5. Place the chocolate into a bowl over a saucepan of boiling water and stir as it melts completely, leave to cool
6. Remove the cookies from the fridge and dip each one into the melted chocolate and place it back onto the tray
7. Pop the tray back into the fridge for a few hours to allow the chocolate to set
8. Pack the cookies away into an airtight container and store in the fridge

Nutritional information:
- **Calories:** 154
- **Fat:** 12.6 grams
- **Protein:** 5 grams
- **Total carbs:** 7.8 grams
- **Net carbs:** 6 grams

Chocolate Avocado Mousse

Avocado makes a perfect base for creamy desserts thanks to its smooth texture and mild taste. We combine avocado, whipped cream and cocoa to create a fat-filled dessert with a good dose of fiber thrown in there too!

Serves: 3
Time: approximately 15 minutes
Ingredients:
- 1 avocado
- 1 cup heavy cream
- 2 Tbsp cocoa powder
- ½ tsp stevia

Method:
1. Place the cream into a bowl and whip until soft and pillowy
2. Transfer the whipped cream into your food processor and add the avocado, cocoa and stevia
3. Blitz the mixture until smooth, soft and creamy
4. Spoon the mousse into three dessert dishes and place into the fridge until needed

Nutritional information:
- **Calories:** 353
- **Fat:** 34.2 grams
- **Protein:** 1.7 grams
- **Total carbs:** 8.2 grams
- **Net carbs:** 3.5 grams

Coconut Vanilla Latte

This hot, creamy latte combines the soft flavors of coconut and vanilla. When you want something decadent, warm and creamy but you don't feel like chocolate…this is your answer.

Serves: 3
Time: 10 minutes
Ingredients:
- 1 cup full-fat coconut cream
- ½ cup heavy cream
- 2 Tbsp vanilla extract
- ½ tsp stevia

Method:
1. Place all ingredients into a saucepan and place over a low heat
2. Stir as the latte becomes hot but doesn't boil or bubble
3. Carefully pour into three mugs before serving

Nutritional information:
- **Calories:** 292
- **Fat:** 26.7 grams
- **Protein:** 1.3 grams
- **Total carbs:** 4.2 grams
- **Net carbs:** 4.2 grams

Peppermint Hot Chocolate

I had to include a peppermint chocolate treat in here somewhere! It's creamy, bitter, refreshing and sweet all at the same time. The perfect way to add more fats to your macros at the end of the day.

Serves: 3
Time: 10 minutes
Ingredients:
- 1 cup heavy cream
- ½ cup almond milk
- 2 Tbsp cocoa powder
- ½ tsp peppermint essence (more or less to taste, just start with a few drops)
- ½ tsp stevia

Method:
1. Place all ingredients into a sauce pan and place over a low heat
2. Whisk as the hot chocolate becomes nice and hot but not bubbling or boiling
3. Carefully pour into three mugs and serve

Nutritional information:
- *Calories:* 280
- *Fat:* 27.6 grams
- *Protein:* 0.9 grams
- *Total carbs:* 4.4 grams
- *Net carbs:* 2.9 grams

Lemon Cream

If there's one thing I actually cannot resist it's a creamy, lemon-flavored dessert! This dessert is stupidly easy. It involves whipped cream, lemon zest, lemon juice and stevia. This dessert is kind of a nod to lemon cream cheese icing and you'll see why...

Serves: 4
Time: approximately 10 minutes plus 30 minutes to chill
Ingredients:
- 1 cup heavy cream
- ½ cup full-fat plain cream cheese, soft
- Juice and zest of 1 juicy lemon
- ½ tsp lemon essence
- ½ tsp stevia

Method:
1. Place the cream into a large bowl and whip until soft and pillowy
2. Add the cream cheese, lemon juice and zest, lemon essence and stevia and whip together until thick and smooth
3. Spoon into four dessert dishes and chill in the fridge for half an hour before serving

Nutritional information:
- **Calories:** 302
- **Fat:** 30 grams
- **Protein:** 1.8 grams
- **Total carbs:** 3.6 grams
- **Net carbs:** 3.6 grams

Sweet and Creamy Chai Latte

We infuse cream and almond milk with tea, spices and stevia to create a warming latte reminiscent of Indian flavors. This is a perfect sweet treat to enjoy after dinner when you don't feel like eating anything but you do feel like slowly sipping away at something hot and sweet.

Serves: 4
Time: 20 minutes
Ingredients:
- 1 cup heavy cream
- 1 cup almond milk
- 2 tea bags (plain tea is fine)
- 1 cinnamon quill
- 4 cloves
- 1 star anise
- 2 cardamom pods
- ½ tsp ground ginger
- ½ tsp stevia

Method:
1. Place all ingredients into a saucepan and place over a low-medium heat and allow the milk to become very hot but not boiling or bubbling
2. Allow the spices to infuse into the cream and almond milk for about 10 minutes
3. Strain the latte through a sieve to catch the tea bags and spices
4. Pour the latte into mugs and serve nice and hot

Nutritional information:
- **Calories:** 208
- **Fat:** 20.6 grams
- **Protein:** 0.3 grams
- **Total carbs:** 1.9 grams
- **Net carbs:** 1.6 grams

Chili Spice Hot Chocolate

In Mexican tradition, chili has been added to hot chocolate drinks for millenia! And it's still popular today, for very good reason. The combination of cocoa and chili is something truly special, and surprisingly invigorating.

Serves: 6 small servings (it's really rich)
Time: approximately 15 minutes
Ingredients:

- 2 oz 72% cocoa dark chocolate
- 2 Tbsp unsweetened cocoa powder
- ½ tsp stevia
- 1 tsp chili powder
- 1 cup heavy cream
- ½ cup almond milk

Method:
1. Place all ingredients into a saucepan and place over a low heat and whisk as the chocolate melts and everything comes together to create a smooth, hot mixture
2. Very carefully pour into four mugs and serve right away
3. Sit around with your loved ones and relax over your spicy, comforting hot chocolate

Nutritional information:

- **Calories:** 193
- **Fat:** 17.5 grams
- **Protein:** 2.1 grams
- **Total carbs:** 7.9 grams
- **Net carbs:** 5.8 grams

Conclusion

Hey there! We got to the end!

By now we are full and satisfied with tasty recipes which will keep us in ketosis without depriving us of flavor and fun.

My wish is that you find these recipes easy to make, time-conscious and above all, yummy. And if something's not working for you in terms of taste preference or sourcing ingredients? Simply change it up! Use your macro tracker to make sure you're still within keto bounds, but go ahead and make these recipes work for *you*.

And hey, keto can be tough for beginners at first. You may feel as though you want to give up and go back to sugar and carbs. But just remember that it's the "keto flu" talking (when your body feels a little odd as it adjusts to the new eating plan). Give yourself a break and get plenty of rest, lighten your load at the gym and drink plenty of water.

I wish you all the luck in the world with your exciting new keto journey!

Made in the USA
Lexington, KY
03 July 2019